foreword

Surf Life Saving Australia is an internationally recognised humanitarian organisation that has been committed to providing a safer community for all Australians for almost one hundred years. It takes a committed individual to undertake first aid training and the decision to do so is not one to be taken lightly. First aid is a major component of all surf lifesaving activities in Australia.

The acquisition of first aid skills places you in a unique position to take responsibility for the health and well-being of your family, community members and workmates, should the need arise. The rewards for you undertaking this training will be the skills and confidence to maybe, one day, save a life.

First aiders are most likely to be the person to respond to an incident. You will be expected to recognise dangers and respond appropriately in a variety of environments and situations. Incidents and environments requiring first aid can range from children in the family home, members of the public involved in a motor vehicle accident to, of course, our beaches. This manual will give you the knowledge to respond to emergency situations with confidence and professionalism.

Our organisation has commissioned professionals from first aid, education and medical services in the development of this manual. Their extensive experience has covered many facets of first aid and emergency care training in this one manual. It is unique in its format, covering basic first aid, senior first aid, triage, oxygen administration, defibrillators, spinal management skills and the administration of analgesic gases. Surf Life Saving Australia has always provided internationally recognised quality training to its members, we are now proud to offer that same training to outside organisations as well.

Lifesaving and education are two aspects of our core business and this manual will help you achieve the skills necessary to serve the public and to be a humanitarian leader in community safety.

Ron Rankin, AM
President
Surf Life Saving Australia

preface

Surf Life Saving Australia has been one of the leading aquatic providers of first aid for nearly one hundred years. Many of the first aid advances in the areas of marine envenomation and resuscitation have been pioneered by Surf Life Saving Australia. The organisation prides itself by articulating first aid as a major component of its core training. Currently, this training is provided to over 100 000 surf lifesavers around the country and also to many members of the public.

First aiders need to know what to do in an emergency before medical assistance arrives. The contents of this manual will equip you with the skills and confidence to act in many emergency situations. Today's first aider is being increasingly trained in smarter technology that is easier to use, often using medical equipment and techniques that, only a decade ago, would be reserved for our hospital emergency wards.

The national competency-based framework demands that teaching organisations produce high quality material while delivering quality-controlled education programs. Surf Life Saving Australia is committed, as a core business outcome, to be a leader in education and training.

This manual is aimed at a number of lifesaving and community groups. It reaches beyond the traditional person on the beach and into our communities, schools, workplaces and families. It integrates best first aid teaching practice from numerous perspectives, providing you with the confidence and skills to be an integral part in a holistic approach to health care in the community.

Thanks to the surf lifesavers and first aid experts who contributed their time and expertise to this project.

Peter George
National Director of Lifesaving
Surf Life Saving Australia

Peter Agnew
National Lifesaving Manager
Surf Life Saving Australia

contents

acknowledgements

This manual is the product of research in the best practice of first aid, drawing on the experience of doctors, paramedics, first aiders and professional educators. It reflects the input of members from all sections of Surf Life Saving Australia (SLSA) and industry.

SLSA acknowledges the many people who have contributed to the preparation and production of this manual, particularly:

The Editorial Panel

Dean Dudley (National Education Co-ordinator to July 2004)

Matthew Lynch (National Education Co-ordinator from July 2004)

Peter George (National Director of Lifesaving)

Peter Agnew (National Lifesaving Manager)

Jenny Kenny (Director of Lifesaving, Tasmania)

Andrew Chubb (Director of Lifesaving, New South Wales)

Dr Peter Fenner (National Medical Advisor)

Craig Roberts (Training and Education Development Officer, SLSQ)

Gary Beauchamp (Sydney Northern Beaches Branch Advanced Lifesaving Supervisor)

John Kitts (SLSWA First Aid Officer)

The National Board of Lifesaving

Peter George (National Director of Lifesaving)

Peter Agnew (National Lifesaving Manager)

Mark Fife (Director of Lifesaving, Queensland)

Andrew Chubb (Director of Lifesaving, New South Wales)

Bob Wood (Director of Lifesaving, Victoria)

Jenny Kenny (Director of Lifesaving, Tasmania)

David Swain (Director of Lifesaving, South Australia)

Tony Snelling (Director of Lifesaving, Western Australia)

Jo Gardiner (Director of Lifesaving, Northern Territory)

Special thanks to

Surf Life Saving Victoria

Steven Faddy, St Vincent's Hospital

Marcia Fife, Surf Life Saving Queensland

Professor John Pearn, Department of Paediatrics and Child Health – Royal Children's Hospital, Brisbane

Danny Chard, Vital Resus

Ambulance Service of New South Wales

Sports Medicine Australia

Australian Resuscitation Council

BOC Medical

The Royal Life Saving Society of Australia

Emergcare — Emergency Care Education Services

Marianne Troop, First Aid Plus, Australia Pty Ltd

DHS Pty Ltd

introduction

formation and foundation of Surf Life Saving Australia

The origins of surf lifesaving can be traced back to the actions of Mr William Gocher who, in September 1902 at Manly Beach, defied the law of the time by bathing during the prohibited daylight hours. His action and similar actions by others forced authorities to confront the issue of daylight bathing as it began to grow rapidly into a national pastime.

As surf bathing became popular, its dangers rapidly became apparent. Small groups of experienced, regular surfers began to form themselves into lifesaving bodies to help people who needed rescuing from an unfamiliar environment.

As these clubs grew in size and number, the need for a united front to raise funds and ask for help from local councils and the New South Wales State Government became apparent. As a result, the New South Wales Surf Bathing Association was formed on 18 October 1907. The name of the association was later changed to The Surf Life Saving Association of Australia and, in 1991, was changed again to Surf Life Saving Australia.

club life and activities

Surf Life Saving Australia (SLSA) has evolved into an organisation known throughout the world for its voluntary humanitarian service. To date, it has performed more than 480 000 recorded rescues.

Outstanding for its feats of courage and reliable service to the surfing public, SLSA continues to be maintained by members who are justly proud of their motto, 'Vigilance and Service'.

Through its affiliated State and Territory centres, branches and clubs, SLSA offers members of the community the opportunity to help in lifesaving work and take part in a nationwide effort that provides valuable rewards and lasting enjoyment.

The comradeship among members, the common participation in a voluntary, humanitarian service, and the many sideline pursuits that form an integral part of surf club activities combine to make SLSA an organisation both unique and necessary to the Australian way of life.

administration of SLSA

Clubs in the two largest lifesaving States, New South Wales and Queensland, are affiliated with a local branch, which is responsible for supervising and controlling patrols, gear, competitions and carnivals, along with determining local policy.

These branches, and the clubs in other States/ Territories, are affiliated with their respective State/ Territory centres. The State/Territory centres are combined into the Australian Council, which is responsible for the administration of the organisation in Australia and its relationship with similar organisations outside Australia.

board of lifesaving

The practical side of surf lifesaving activities is controlled by the Board of Lifesaving in each branch and State/Territory centre. These dedicated groups of lifesavers carry out various duties including conducting assessments, supervising and instructing awards, inspecting equipment, overseeing beach patrols and conducting annual surf lifesaver proficiency tests.

Representatives of the boards meet on a branch and State/Territory basis as well as on a national basis, at regular lifesaving conferences, and submit recommendations on surf lifesaving procedures and practices to the Australian Council. If approved, these practices are incorporated into the manuals of Surf Life Saving Australia. This manual incorporates several SLSA endorsed awards including Senior First Aid Certificate, Advanced Resuscitation Certificate, Defibrillation Certificate and the Silver Medallion (Advanced Emergency Care).

international lifesaving

In November 1956, the Australian Council of SLSA joined with the Surf Life Saving Associations of New Zealand, South Africa, Ceylon, Hawaii, Great Britain and the USA to establish the International Council of Surf Life Saving, with headquarters in Toronto, Canada.

In 1971, after a meeting in Sydney, all affiliates to the International Council of Surf Life Saving joined to form a new, fully constituted organisation called World Life Saving.

In 1993, World Life Saving (WLS) and The Fédération Internationale de Sauvetage Aquatique (FIS) united to become the International Life Saving Federation (ILS), with headquarters in Leuven, Belgium. This worldwide organisation co-ordinates the activities of the rescue, education, medical and competition committees, for the benefit of all member nations.

the Australian Qualifications Framework

The Australian Qualifications Framework (AQF) provides a national framework for all education and training qualifications. The aim of the AQF is to:

+ provide consistent qualifications
+ encourage easier access to qualifications
+ provide flexible pathways for achieving qualifications.

The AQF covers qualifications issued by the secondary schools sector, vocational education and training (VET) sector and the higher education sector. Under the AQF, qualifications issued in the VET sector are based on the achievement of competency standards.

The qualifications within each sector are shown below.

The public safety industry comprises organisations such as the Police Force, Fire Brigade, State and Territory Emergency Services, Emergency Management Sectors and Surf Life Saving Australia.

The public safety industry generally follows a number of key principles and requirements such as the following:

+ assessment and appeals
+ recognition of prior learning (RPL)
+ equal employment opportunities
+ harassment-free workplace
+ limiting and permanent disability.

recognition of prior learning

You may already have some skills for the courses in this manual. Perhaps you completed similar activities in previous work or learned them in another training course.

If you can demonstrate to your training officer that you are competent in a particular skill, you may not need to repeat the training for that skill. This is called RPL, which stands for 'recognition of prior learning'. It is also known as RCC (recognition of current competency). Your prior learning is recognised when you can successfully demonstrate that you are competent in a particular skill. Some skills may need to be articulated into a first-aid environment and you will also need to demonstrate your ability to achieve this.

If you feel that you have some relevant skills, talk to your training officer about having them formally recognised. Your training officer will then check to make sure you can do all the required activities and advise you of the formal process needed to be undertaken for RPL.

AQF QUALIFICATIONS BY SECTOR

SCHOOL SECTOR	VOCATIONAL EDUCATION AND TRAINING SECTOR	HIGHER EDUCATION SECTOR
		Doctoral Degree
		Masters Degree
		Graduate Diploma
		Graduate Certificate
		Bachelor Degree
	Advanced Diploma	Advanced Diploma
	Diploma	Diploma
	Certificate IV	
	Certificate III	
Senior Secondary	Certificate II	
Certificate of	Certificate I	
Education		

introduction to first aid

learning outcomes

Identify the underpinning context and safety requirements for first aid and emergency care using approved SLSA procedures.

+ Detail the aims of first aid and emergency care.
+ Describe the causes of accidents and illnesses.
+ Detail the principles of occupational health and safety as they apply to first aid and emergency care.
+ Detail legal aspects that apply to first aid and emergency care.
+ Describe the process for documenting first aid incidents and treatments.
+ Detail the contents and maintenance of first aid kits and first aid rooms.
+ Describe the types and specific application of personal protection equipment.
+ Detail the protocols for the management of blood and body-substance spills.

how you may be assessed

underpinning knowledge

A number of oral or written questions may be asked relating to the aims of first aid and emergency care, the causes of accidents and illnesses, occupational health and safety, legal aspects of first aid, documenting first aid treatments and incidents, first aid kits and rooms, personal protection equipment and blood and body-substance spills. Examples have been included at the end of the chapter.

practical demonstration

You may be asked to show how you would document first aid incidents and treatments using the correct forms and procedures. You may be asked to show the location of first aid kits and describe their contents. You may be required to identify the contents of a first aid room. You may be required to demonstrate the use of personal protection equipment during first aid treatments.

scenario

You may be required to locate a first aid kit, use personal protective equipment and correctly document any first aid treatments and incidents.

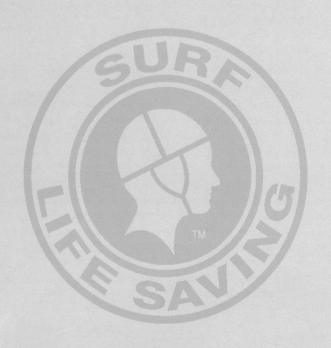

what is first aid?

First aid is the immediate or emergency assistance given on the spot to people suffering from illness or injury.

First aid knowledge and skills are invaluable. Emergencies can happen at any time and someone equipped with sufficient first aid knowledge, skills and confidence can make the difference between life and death for a sick or injured person. Many people save family members, friends and strangers by using the simple first aid skills they have acquired through first aid training.

aims of first aid

The aims of first aid are to:

✚ *provide* reassurance and comfort to the ill or injured
✚ *prevent* injury or illness becoming worse (cause no harm)
✚ *protect* the unconscious patient
✚ *preserve* life
✚ *promote* recovery

causes of accidents and illness

First aid training is of particular use in the workplace. Unsafe working conditions and practices can lead to injury, illness or even death. Anything that places a person at risk is a hazard.

Some hazards may not be obvious, such as poisonous gases or poorly stored fuel.

code of practice

Codes of practice are designed to provide practical guidance to employers, employees and self-employed people, and each State implements a code of practice that adopts these principles.

The First Aid Code of Practice provides practical guidance in the provision of emergency treatment and life-support procedures for people suffering illness or injury at work.

The First Aid Code of Practice provides guidelines for employers, in consultation with first aiders, elected health and safety representatives and employees, to assess their workplace to determine what first aid facilities and training are required.

Depending on the size of the workplace, number of employees and perceived risks to health and safety, the number of first aiders and the equipment required will vary from a single first aider with a basic kit to a designated medical room with a full-time nurse and a staff of first aiders.

People may also create hazards by careless mistakes or practical jokes, often contributing to personal injury.

Some potential hazards in the workplace are described below. This list is not exhaustive, and many other things may cause accidents or injury in the workplace. As first aiders, we should all act responsibly and seek to prevent accidents by paying attention to things that could be hazardous and removing those risks.

All accidents and incidents must be reported to an appropriate supervisor, and logged in an Incident Log Book or other appropriate record document. All accidents outside work hours, but on work premises, should also be recorded.

potential hazards in the workplace

obstructions

Spare equipment piled in fire exits or stairwells may obstruct you from being able to obtain rescue equipment, thereby delaying your response to an incident.

spills and slippery surfaces

A simple spill of water, food, oils, boat fuel or any other substance on the floor may be hazardous. Rock surfaces and pool walkways may also be slippery and hazardous.

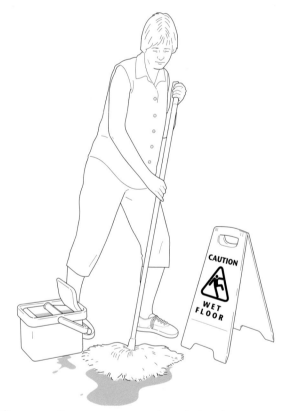

Slippery surfaces are a potential workplace hazard

faulty maintenance

Damaged rescue boards or equipment, broken propeller guards on inflatable rescue boat (IRB) motors, or a patrol enclosure in disrepair are all examples of hazards. All breakdowns and faulty equipment must be reported and must be repaired by a qualified person.

environmental causes

Sun exposure is a potential hazard associated with long periods of time spent working outdoors. Adequate clothing and sun protection are essential to avoid skin damage. The ocean environment also creates a unique blend of hazards in the form of waves, shallow water and rips.

incorrect storage

Incorrect storage of any item is a hazard. When storing or stacking things away, heavy items should be placed on the bottom, with lighter items on top. Fuel and chemicals should always be stored separately in well ventilated, cool areas. This prevents fumes building up and avoids explosions if the chemicals react to heat. Flammable materials have specific storage requirements. Storage areas should have strong shelves suitable for the material to be stored. Milk crates and boxes are not shelves and should not be used as such.

incorrect use of equipment

Rescue equipment and other specialised equipment should always be used by qualified members and in designated areas. Training areas should be set up with adequate signage and in an area that will not cause harm to the public.

lifting and carrying

Moving and carrying equipment is a necessary component of the role of lifesavers and first aiders. To prevent back injury, correct posture should be assumed at all times when lifting. Wherever possible, heavy items should be carried on a trolley or with the assistance of others. The lifting of people needs to be conducted in a safe manner. The use of team carries and stretchers is strongly recommended.

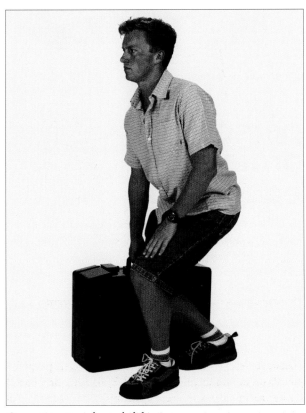

Correct posture for safe lifting

infection

Barrier methods of protection, such as gloves and masks are essential to protect the patient and first aider from the spread of infectious diseases. These methods should be used routinely, especially during resuscitation or when exposed to blood or other body fluids.

occupational health and safety

Commonwealth and State occupational/workplace health and safety legislation places a duty on employers to provide information, instruction, training and supervision to employees to enable them to perform their work in a safe manner without risk to health.

first aid and the law

consent

All patients have the right to accept or refuse treatment. There are two kinds of consent:

+ *actual consent:* the patient/guardian gives a first aider permission to help them/their charge or apply first aid
+ *implied consent:* in an emergency situation, the consent of the unconscious person or parent/guardian of a child is implicit.

duty of care

Australian law does not impose a duty of care on any person to give assistance unless that person already owes a duty of care to the sick or injured person.

A first aider at a work site has an implied duty of care, as does someone caring for children. There is no such *clear* duty for a volunteer, but once a person starts to act, that person becomes the caregiver and should stay with the sick or injured person until professional help arrives.

negligence

In the event of a negligence action, a court has to be persuaded by the plaintiff that the damage was caused by a first aider's negligence.

Negligence is established only if all of the following are found:

+ the first aider owed a duty of care to the injured person and the standard of care required by that duty was breached
+ damage was caused by the breach of the duty of care
+ the event was reasonably foreseeable.

protection against litigation

First aiders will be judged by the standard of first aid to which they have been trained. The court must prove that damage was caused by their negligence, as outlined above.

You can protect yourself against litigation by:

✚ following guidelines as set down in this and other accepted manuals
✚ doing your best to assess priorities of care
✚ stabilising the patient until professional help arrives
✚ keeping accurate and detailed records of first aid care given.

documenting first aid incidents

Documentation of all incidents and all patients managed by first aiders is essential. It provides protection for the injured person, the first aider and, if in the workplace, the employer.

Written documentation is mandatory under State regulations for occupational health and safety, and can be used to support insurance, compensation or workers compensation claims.

Continuing documentation of injuries allows for the collection of data on hazards within a workplace and helps first aiders provide the best possible care for the types of injuries likely to be sustained.

✚ All documentation needs to be accurate and legible.
✚ Record only the actual events you witnessed. Record only the facts, not hearsay.
✚ All records should be written in ink. Any mistakes should have a line ruled through them and marked 'wrong entry'. Never erase a mistake or use correction fluid.
✚ All records should be signed by the first aider.
✚ Records should be kept on file in line with the organisation's policies and procedures.

NOTE:
Many organisations have specific first aid reporting documentation that should be completed. See Appendix 1.

first aid kit contents

Various State regulations may stipulate appropriate contents of a first aid kit. See Appendix 2 for an example.

maintaining the first aid kit

First aid equipment should be replaced after use so that a first aid kit is always fully stocked and ready for use. There are a number of points to consider in relation to maintaining first aid equipment:

✚ make sure that first aid kits and equipment are checked regularly
✚ restock first aid supplies after use or prior to expiry
✚ clean equipment after use
✚ develop and implement protocols to ensure first aid equipment is ready for use at all times
✚ record any discrepancies, using established protocols.

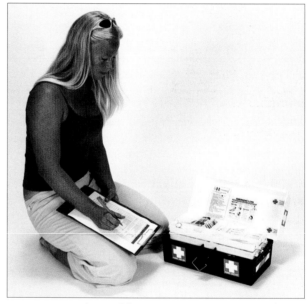
Maintaining a first aid kit

personal protection equipment

First aiders should ensure their personal safety by adequate personal protection against infection. The prevalence of hepatitis B, HIV and other infections in the community has highlighted the need for greater care when providing first aid or resuscitation.

First aiders can protect themselves from infection in a number of ways and still be able to help an injured or ill person.

The three lines of defence for first aiders are:

✚ immunisation
✚ barrier methods
✚ hygiene.

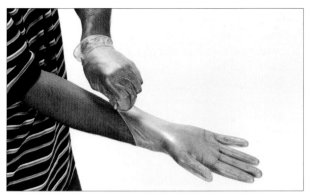

Gloves are an important component of personal protection

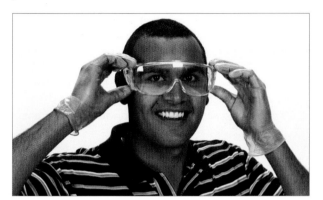

Protective goggles are an important component of personal protection

immunisation

Immunisation is acquiring specific immunity against a disease through vaccination.

Immunisation may help when the other lines of defence are broken. For example, a sharp item such as a needle or piece of glass may cut through a protective glove and the skin, leaving the body open to infection: immunisation will help the body defend itself against associated disease.

As a minimum requirement, Surf Life Saving Australia (SLSA) recommends that first aiders be immunised against hepatitis B and tetanus. First aiders should be encouraged to seek more information on immunisation from a health care professional.

barrier methods

Barrier methods of protection are an easy and essential line of defence against infections. First aiders must avoid direct contact with the blood and other body substances of the person being treated. For your own safety, SLSA strongly recommends that you wear protective clothing when dealing with first aid cases. Latex gloves (or if allergic to latex, vinyl or nitrile) are a simple and effective means of protecting your skin from direct contact with potentially infectious body fluids. Other protective clothing includes safety glasses, facemasks, plastic aprons and appropriate footwear.

hygiene

The third line of defence is hygiene — washing hands thoroughly before and after touching a patient, keeping fingernails short and practising good personal hygiene can help prevent cross-infection.

Any contaminated area should be scrubbed with hot water and soap or detergent for 2 minutes. If you are not immunised against hepatitis B, or if the patient is suspected to have other communicable diseases, you should see a doctor as soon as is reasonably possible.

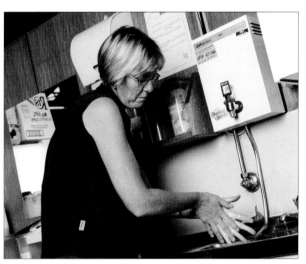

Wash hands thoroughly before and after contact with each patient

NOTE:
- Immunoglobulin for hepatitis B administered within 72 hours of suspected infection is effective in the prevention of the development of hepatitis B.
- See SLSA's Hepatitis Vaccinations Policy or appropriate policies for the workplace at www.slsa.asn.au.

cleaning of first aid rooms

Hygiene also relates to equipment and first aid rooms, which must be kept clean at all times.

The following cleaning recommendations have been adapted from the *Infection Control Guidelines for the Prevention of Transmission of Infectious Diseases in the Health Care Setting* by the Communicable Diseases Network Australia (September 2002).

routine surface cleaning

✚ Written cleaning protocols should be prepared, including methods and frequency of cleaning.

+ Standard precautions (including wearing of personal protective equipment, as appropriate) should be taken when cleaning surfaces and facilities.
+ Work surfaces should be cleaned and dried before use, after use, and when visibly soiled.
+ A solution of detergent (disinfectant or antibacterial solution) and hot water should be used for all routine and general cleaning.
+ Buckets and mops should be washed with detergent and hot water, then stored dry.
+ Cleaning items (including solutions, water, buckets, cleaning cloths and mop heads) should be changed regularly. They should also be changed immediately following the cleaning of blood or body-substance spills.

management of spills

+ Written protocols for dealing with blood and body-substance spills should be included in procedural manuals and emphasised in ongoing education and training programs.
+ Spills should be cleared up before the area is cleaned (adding cleaning liquids to spills increases the size of the spill). Generation of fumes from spilled material should be avoided. It is generally unnecessary to use bleach (sodium hypochlorite) for managing spills.
+ Waste matter contaminated by blood or other body fluids must be placed in separate waste bins lined with 'Hazard Waste' polythene bags. These bags must be separately disposed of within local health authority laws.

small spills

+ Wearing gloves, wipe up spots or drops of blood or other small spills immediately with paper towelling.
+ Clean the area with detergent and hot water.

large spills

+ Chlorine granules can be used to contain and disinfect the spilled material.
+ A scraper and pan should be used to remove the absorbed material.
+ The area should then be cleaned with hot water and detergent using a mop.
+ The mop and bucket should be thoroughly cleaned after use and stored dry.
+ Standard cleaning equipment, including a mop and cleaning bucket plus cleaning agents, should be readily available for spills management and stored in an area known to all personnel.

---

spills kit

To help manage spills in areas where cleaning materials may not be readily available, it is advisable to have a portable 'spills kit' consisting of a large (10 L) plastic container or bucket with fitted lid, containing the following items:

+ disposable rubber gloves
+ appropriate leak-proof bags and containers for disposal of waste material (disposable)
+ a designated sturdy scraper and pan for spills (similar to a 'pooper scooper')
+ about five sachets of a granular (chlorine-releasing) disinfectant formulation containing 10 000 parts per million available chlorine or equivalent (each sachet should contain sufficient granules to cover a spill of 10 cm in diameter)
+ eye protection (disposable or reusable)
+ a plastic apron.

Disposable items in the spills kit should be replaced after each use. With all spills management protocols, it is essential that the affected area is left clean and dry.

revision

1. Which of the following is *not* an aim of first aid?
   a) To provide reassurance and comfort to the ill or injured.
   b) To prevent injury or illness becoming worse (cause no harm).
   c) To protect the conscious patient before the unconscious patient.
   d) To preserve life.

2. What should be recorded in the Incident Log Book?

   _____

   _____

   _____

3. Compete the following sentence as it relates to occupational health and safety.

   Commonwealth and State occupational/workplace health and safety legislation places a duty on employers to

   provide ...., instruction, ... and supervision to employees to enable them to perform their

   work in a safe manner without risk to ....

4. List five potential hazards in the workplace
   a) _____   b) _____   c) _____
   d) _____   e) _____

5. All patients have the right to accept or refuse treatment. What are the two kinds of patient consent?
   a) _____   b) _____

6. List the three lines of defence the first aider should take against infection:
   a) _____   b) _____   c) _____

7. In the event of a negligence action, a first aider's negligence is established by which three criteria?
   a) _____
   b) _____
   c) _____

8. Why should all first aid incidents be documented?

   _____

   _____

   _____

Answers appear in Appendix 8.

anatomy and physiology

learning outcomes

Use correct anatomical terminology required for first aid and emergency care.

+ Describe the position and components of body structures and systems.
+ Detail the relationships between various body structures and systems.
+ Describe the sites of injuries using correct anatomical terminology.

how you may be assessed

underpinning knowledge

A number of oral or written questions may be asked relating to body structures and systems requiring the correct use of anatomical terminology. Examples have been included at the end of the chapter.

practical demonstration

You may be asked to explain the relationships between body structures and systems. You may be asked to show the sites of injuries using correct anatomical terminology.

scenario

You may be required to identify the sites of injuries on a patient using correct anatomical terminology.

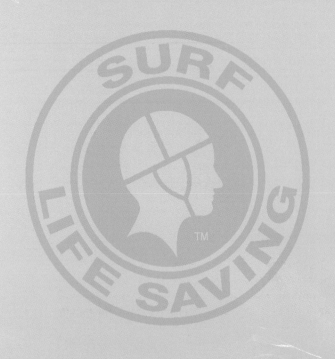

anatomical terminology

Descriptive terminology is necessary to describe the position and relationship of different structures to each other without ambiguity. It is necessary to be familiar with some anatomical terminology to be able to accurately describe body structures and sites of injury. Information on the position and relationship of body structures to each other can be found in Appendix 3.

musculoskeletal system

The skeletal system consists of a rigid framework of bones (206 in the adult) called the skeleton. Bones perform many functions. They:

+ provide structural support for the body
+ protect vital body organs (e.g. brain, heart, lungs)
+ provide an anchor for muscle tendons, allowing joint movement
+ are an important site for the production of blood
+ provide a mineral (e.g. calcium) reservoir for the body.

The bones of the skeleton are connected by a series of joints. Some joints permit virtually no movement, e.g. the bones of the skull, while others are designed to permit movement, e.g. the shoulder, elbow, hip, and knee joints. Joints are held in place by fibrous bands called ligaments. Generally, the greater the range of movement, the less stable the joint, so the shoulder joint, which allows a great range of movement, is prone to dislocation.

Muscles attach to bones via tendons. Contraction and relaxation of muscle allows movement of the bones, thereby enabling the body to move.

The skeleton consists of the:

+ skull, which encloses and protects the brain. The lower jaw, or mandible, articulates with the skull
+ backbone, or vertebral column, which encloses and protects the spinal cord
+ rib cage, which protects the lungs and heart
+ bones of the upper limbs
+ pelvis (hip)
+ bones of the lower limbs.

The most common injuries seen by first aiders are:

+ sprains (overstretched ligaments)
+ strains (overstretched muscles and tendons)
+ fractures (broken bones)
+ dislocations (disarticulated joints).

The vertebral column (spine) is composed of 33 individual bones (vertebrae) separated by softer connective tissue discs and supported by strong ligaments. The spine's structure provides a partly rigid and partly flexible axis for the body and protects the delicate spinal cord.

The spine has an important role in posture and supporting body weight (transferring it to the hips and legs). The spinal column is divided into five sections, three of which are mobile:

+ cervical spine (neck)
+ thoracic spine (thorax or mid-back)
+ lumbar spine (lower back).

The immobile sections are the sacrum (the posterior wall of the pelvis) and the coccyx (tail bone). It takes a considerable amount of force to damage both the spinal column and the spinal cord. The cervical spine, however, is particularly vulnerable because of the:

+ narrow canal in which the spinal cord is contained within the cervical vertebrae
+ lack of extra support, e.g. from bones such as the ribs or pelvis, etc
+ force that the heavy head and brain exert on the cervical spine, particularly in acceleration and deceleration injuries (e.g. the violent forward and backward movement of the head and neck, as in 'whiplash' injuries).

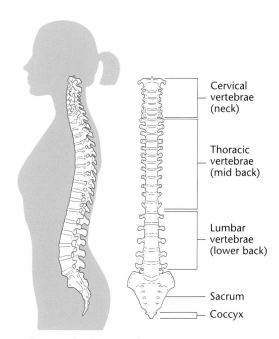

The spinal column — lateral and posterior view

respiratory system

The respiratory system consists of upper and lower tracts. A clear, open airway is the single most important factor for successful resuscitation.

upper respiratory tract

The upper respiratory tract includes the nostrils, nasal cavity, mouth, pharynx (throat) and larynx (voice box).

The throat is a common passageway for both food and air. It starts from the cavity at the back of the mouth

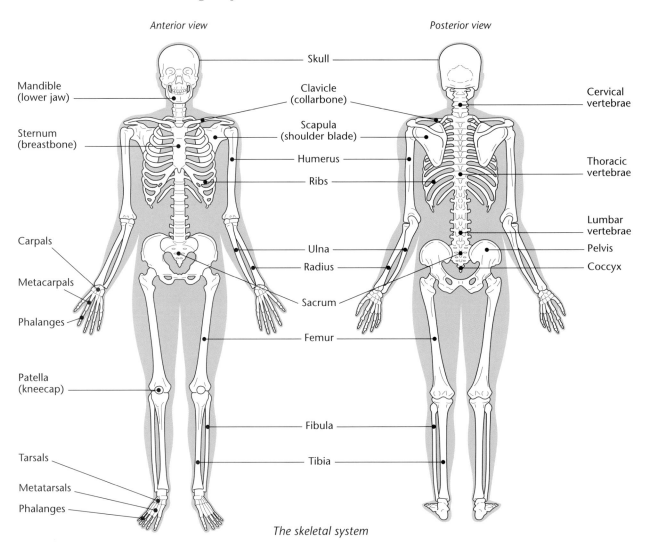

The skeletal system

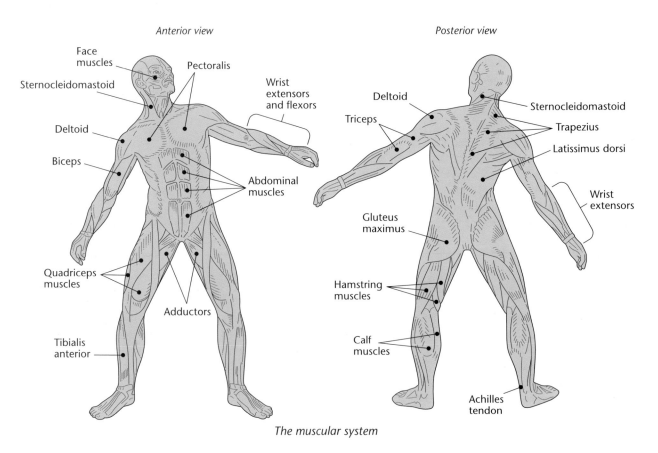

The muscular system

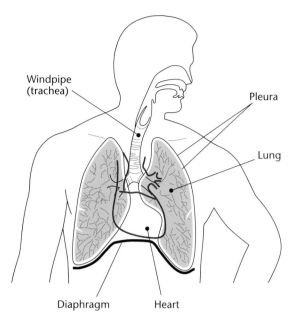

The respiratory system

and nose (the oropharynx) and extends down to where it divides into two separate tubes. The trachea (windpipe), allows the passage of air to and from the lungs. It sits in the front (anteriorly) of the throat and begins at the larynx and vocal cords, extending down toward the lungs. The oesophagus, sits behind (posteriorly) the trachea and carries food and liquids to the stomach (or back from the stomach to the throat during vomiting or regurgitation).

lower respiratory tract

The lower respiratory tract consists of the trachea and the bronchi, which divide into two to enter the right and left lung. The primary bronchi then divide into progressively smaller bronchi, bronchioles and, finally, alveoli (terminal air sacs). The trachea and bronchi are kept open by C-shaped rings of strong connective tissue (cartilage), making them semi-rigid tubes (rather like the vacuum tubing used to clean out swimming pools). These rings hold open the trachea and bronchi, allowing airflow to and from the lungs.

The lungs fill most of the chest cavity, which is separated from the abdomen by a large sheet of muscle known as the diaphragm. The lungs are spongy, elastic organs consisting of the bronchial tree, alveoli (air sacs) and blood vessels.

When we breathe in, air containing oxygen moves (diffuses) into the lungs through to the alveoli. The alveoli are surrounded by tiny blood vessels (capillaries). The interface between these two structures is known as the respiratory membrane, and it allows the exchange (diffusion) of gases. Oxygen diffuses from the alveoli into the blood in the capillaries, while carbon dioxide diffuses from the blood to the alveoli. Carbon dioxide is a waste product of metabolism (burning of the body's energy systems) and is expelled as we breathe out.

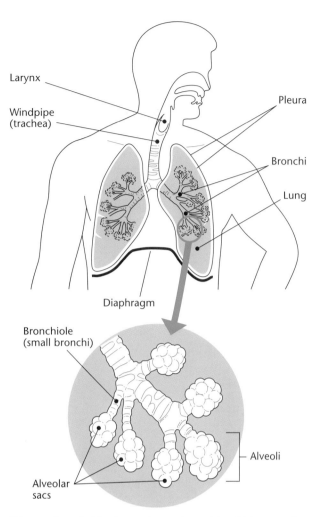

The trachea divides into primary bronchi, which enter the lungs to branch into progressively smaller tubes, ending in alveoli

breathing

Breathing is the act of moving air into and out of the lungs.

Inspiration is the breath in. It is an involuntary muscular action caused by contraction of the muscles that lift the ribs while the diaphragm is pulled down and flattened. This combined action increases the size of the chest cavity and sucks air into the lungs.

Expiration is the breath out. When the muscles of inspiration relax, the elastic recoil of the lung tissues pushes air out of the lungs.

The air we breathe in contains approximately 21% oxygen. About 5% of this is used in the body, so the air we breathe out contains 16% oxygen.

On average, an adult takes about 12–15 breaths per minute. The average amount of air taken in one breath is about half a litre, and is called the tidal volume. In children and infants, the breathing rate is faster and the tidal volume is smaller.

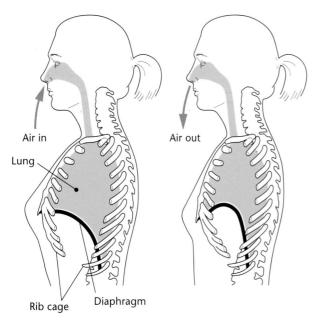

Air in

Lung

Rib cage   Diaphragm

A side (lateral) view of the respiratory system during inspiration and expiration

Air out

breathing control centre

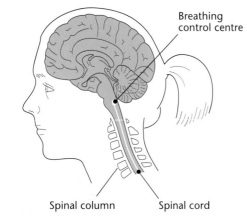

Breathing control centre

Spinal column   Spinal cord

The breathing control centre is located in the brainstem

The breathing control centre is located at the base of the brain in the brainstem. It acts like a metronome (timing mechanism), sending out regular impulses that control the rate and depth of breathing (both inspiration and expiration). The breathing control centre must have a good supply of oxygen, otherwise this nervous tissue will become damaged and not function properly and breathing will stop.

circulatory system

The circulatory system consists of the heart and blood vessels. The heart is a muscular pump, about the size of a clenched fist. It has four chambers:

✚ two atria, which receive blood to pump to the ventricles
✚ two ventricles, one that pumps blood to the lungs (right), and another that pumps blood to the body (left).

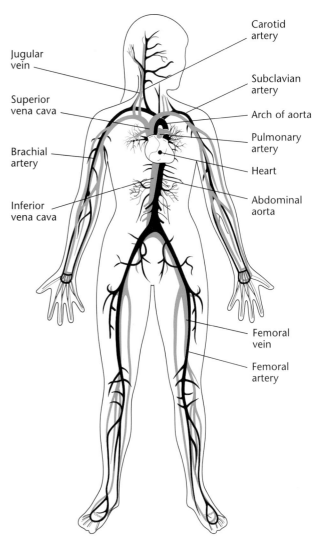

Jugular vein

Superior vena cava

Brachial artery

Inferior vena cava

Carotid artery

Subclavian artery

Arch of aorta

Pulmonary artery

Heart

Abdominal aorta

Femoral vein

Femoral artery

The circulatory system. The right side of the heart and veins contain deoxygenated blood and are shown in blue and the left side of the heart and arteries contain oxygenated blood (except the pulmonary artery) and are shown in red

The right side of the heart receives deoxygenated or venous blood from veins throughout the body and pumps blood to the lungs. The left side of the heart receives oxygenated blood from the lungs and pumps it throughout the body's arteries via the aorta (main output tract of the heart).

Arteries circulate blood at high pressure, so their walls are thick and muscular. Major arteries are often located deep within the body tissue. Arterial blood is bright red due to its oxygen content. Serious blood loss can occur rapidly when someone is bleeding from an artery, because of the high blood pressure, which causes the escaping blood to spurt in time with the heartbeat. Arterial bleeding is unlikely to stop of its own accord.

Veins circulate blood at low pressure, so their walls are thin. Veins contain valves that prevent the backflow of blood. Many veins are located close to the skin (superficially), such as those visible under the skin on the feet, hands and forearms. Venous blood is dark red, due to its low oxygen content.

Capillaries are the smallest blood vessels and capillary networks link the ends of the smallest arteries with the smallest veins. Capillaries allow oxygen and nutrients to

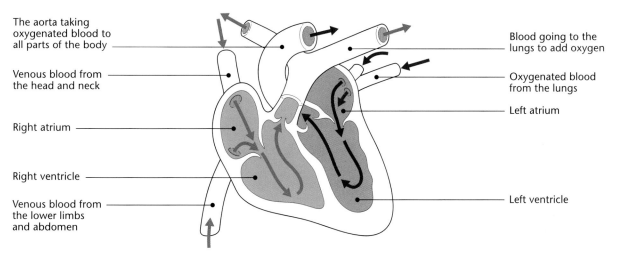

The aorta taking oxygenated blood to all parts of the body

Venous blood from the head and neck

Right atrium

Right ventricle

Venous blood from the lower limbs and abdomen

Blood going to the lungs to add oxygen

Oxygenated blood from the lungs

Left atrium

Left ventricle

Anatomy of the heart. The direction of blood flow is indicated by arrows, with red arrows representing oxygenated blood and blue arrows indicating deoxygenated blood

reach every cell in the body, and carbon dioxide and other waste products to be removed.

With the exception of the fingernails, toenails and hair, injury to any part of the body will cause damage to blood vessels, and result in some degree of bleeding (from minor bruising to major life-threatening bleeds).

For the organs and all parts of the body to receive adequate oxygen, normal heart function is essential to oxygenate blood and pump it throughout the body. When the heart stops, oxygen is not supplied to the body. The brain is highly susceptible to lack of oxygen (hypoxia) and damage may occur if blood supply is not restored within 3–5 minutes.

pulse

When a first aider checks a pulse, they are feeling an artery pulsating with each contraction of the heart.

The major sites to feel the pulse are the:

+ carotid artery in the neck
+ brachial artery just above the elbow (mainly felt in infants)
+ radial artery at the wrist
+ femoral artery in the groin.

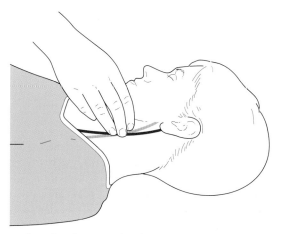

Feeling for the carotid pulse

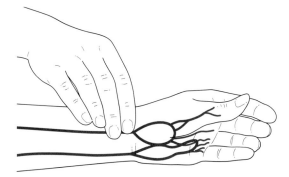

Feeling for the radial pulse

lymphatic system

The lymphatic system mainly comprises the lymph glands and lymph vessels. The tonsils, spleen and thymus gland also form part of the lymphatic system, as do lymphocytes (white blood cells). The functions of the lymphatic system are to:

+ maintain tissue fluid balance. Fluid seeps out of capillaries each day, and enters the lymphatic system, where it is referred to as lymph. Lymph is returned back to the circulatory system
+ absorb fats and other substances from the digestive system
+ assist immunity (the body's defence system). Lymphocytes are produced in the lymphatic system. Lymph is filtered through nodes and the spleen to remove 'foreign' material (antigens) and lymphocytes produce antibodies that can destroy 'foreign' protein matter (e.g. bacteria).

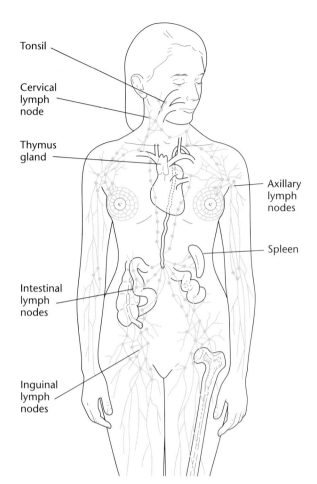

Tonsil

Cervical
lymph
node

Thymus
gland

Axillary
lymph
nodes

Spleen

Intestinal
lymph
nodes

Inguinal
lymph
nodes

The lymphatic system

nervous system

The nervous system comprises central and peripheral divisions that work together to regulate and co-ordinate all body systems.

central nervous system

The brain and spinal cord comprise the central nervous system.

The brain is divided into the:

+ *brainstem*: responsible for basic life-support functions, including the heartbeat and respiration
+ *cerebellum*: involved in motor control, muscle co-ordination and muscle tone
+ *cerebral hemispheres*: the largest part of the brain and responsible for all other functions, movement, senses, memory and higher cognitive function.

Messages from the brain are relayed throughout the body via the spinal cord and a complex network of nerve pathways, which extends throughout the entire body.

Brain cells require a continuous supply of oxygen in order to function. Irreversible damage can occur if brain cells are starved of oxygen for more than 3–5 minutes.

peripheral nervous system

The peripheral nervous system constitutes all the nerves, ganglia (clusters of nerve cell bodies) and sensory recep-

tors outside the central nervous system. It includes the somatic system, which relays impulses from the central nervous system to voluntary muscles (skeletal muscle) as well as an autonomic system, which relays impulses from the central nervous system to involuntary muscles (cardiac muscle and smooth muscle, e.g. around blood vessels) and glands.

The autonomic nervous system has sympathetic and parasympathetic divisions:

+ the sympathetic nervous system is responsible for the 'fight or flight' response to emergency or stressful situations (release of adrenaline causes increased heart rate and blood pressure and diverts blood away from visceral organs [e.g. stomach, intestines] to the brain and skeletal muscle)
+ the parasympathetic nervous system acts to restore and conserve body systems.

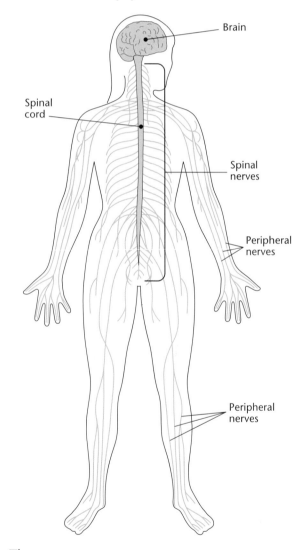

Brain

Spinal
cord

Spinal
nerves

Peripheral
nerves

Peripheral
nerves

The nervous system

digestive system

Food is essential for providing all the nutrients and energy required for our body cells to function properly. The digestive system is responsible for breaking down and processing the food we eat (digestion) so that nutrients can be transported to the cells for production of energy. It is also responsible for eliminating waste products from the digestive process.

The major organs in the digestive system are the:

➕ mouth (including the salivary glands and tonsils)
➕ oesophagus
➕ stomach
➕ liver
➕ gall bladder
➕ pancreas
➕ duodenum
➕ small intestine
➕ large intestine
➕ rectum (terminating at the anus).

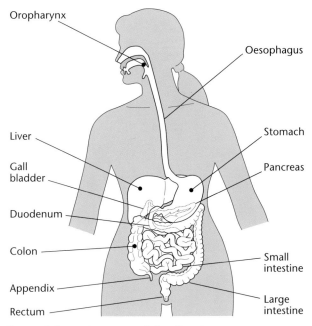

Some of the main organs of the digestive system

integumentary system (skin)

The skin is the outermost layer that protects and covers the entire body. It consists of three layers, the dermis, the epidermis and the underlying hypodermis containing nerves, blood vessels and fat (adipose) tissue. Its functions are to:

➕ protect the underlying tissues and organs
➕ prevent the entry of infectious agents (first line of defence)

➕ maintain and regulate body temperature
➕ prevent dehydration
➕ detect stimuli (e.g. touch, pressure, vibration, pain)
➕ provide a factory for vitamin D production and storage (necessary for strong bones).

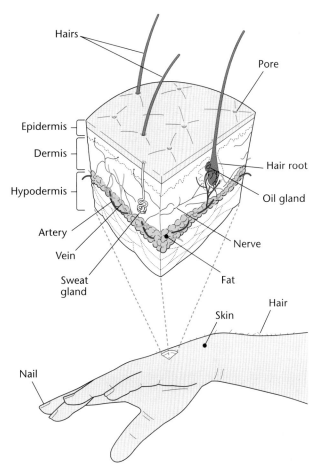

Cross-section of skin

urinary system

The urinary system helps rid the body of waste products. It does this by filtering blood through the kidneys, regulating fluid and chemical (electrolyte) balance, excreting or reabsorbing substances as required. From the kidneys, urine drains down the ureters into the bladder and is then passed out of the body via the urethra.

The kidneys filter approximately 125 mL of blood per minute. An average adult produces about 1–2 L of urine per day, depending on fluid intake, temperature, blood pressure and general health. The kidneys also play a major role in regulating blood volume and blood pH (acidity/alkalinity).

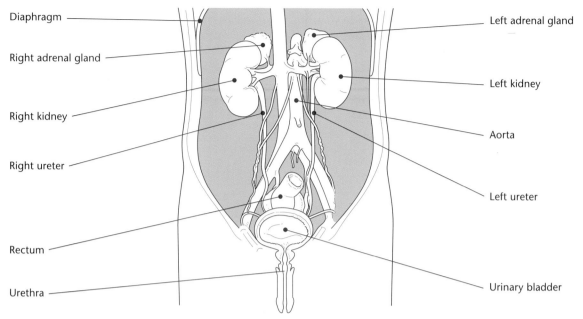

Diaphragm

Right adrenal gland

Right kidney

Right ureter

Rectum

Urethra

Left adrenal gland

Left kidney

Aorta

Left ureter

Urinary bladder

The urinary system

endocrine system

The endocrine system helps regulate and co-ordinate bodily functions and structures. It consists of glands that secrete hormones into the circulatory system, where they act on specific tissues or organs. Endocrine glands include the following:

+ *pituitary gland*: located in the brain, it is responsible for the efficient functioning of all the other endocrine glands
+ *thyroid*: located in the front of the throat, it is responsible for the 'speed' at which the body works (basal metabolic rate, i.e. normal, over-active or under-active) and calcium metabolism (important for bone strength)
+ *adrenal glands*: located on top of the kidneys, they control the main body functions
+ *pancreas*: located deep in the upper part of the abdomen under the stomach, it is responsible for producing insulin (regulates blood sugar level)
+ *ovaries* (females) and *testes* (males): responsible for the production of sex hormones, sexual development and function (sperm production in men, and menstruation and pregnancy in women).

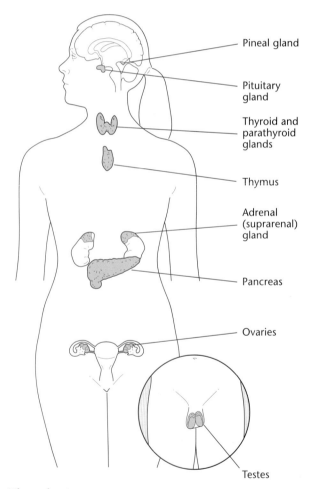

Pineal gland

Pituitary gland

Thyroid and parathyroid glands

Thymus

Adrenal (suprarenal) gland

Pancreas

Ovaries

Testes

The endocrine system

revision

1. Why is descriptive anatomical terminology necessary in first aid?

   _____

   _____

2. What are the most common musculoskeletal injuries likely to be seen by the first aider?

   a) _____   b) _____

   c) _____   d) _____

3. List the components of the upper respiratory tract.

   _____

   _____

4. List the components of the lower respiratory tract.

   _____

   _____

5. Complete the following sentence.

   The heart has four chambers, two ...., which .... blood to pump to the ventricles, and two

   ventricles, one that pumps blood to the .... (right), and another that pumps blood to the body

   (.................).

6. List the four major sites the first aider may feel a pulse:

   a) _____

   b) _____

   c) _____

   d) _____

7. List the three functions of the lymphatic system:

   a) _____

   b) _____

   c) _____

8. What are the major components of the brain and what functions are they involved with?

   a) _____

   b) _____

   c) _____

9. List the two layers of the skin:

   a) _____   b) _____

10. Which of the following features of the kidney is *not* true?
    a) Kidneys filter blood.   b) Kidneys regulate blood volume.
    c) Kidneys regulate blood pH.   d) Kidneys produce 3–4 L of urine per day.

Answers appear in Appendix 8.

first aid management

learning outcomes

Perform basic life support practices and correct first aid incident management.

+ Describe the basic principles of first aid incident management.
+ Detail basic life support including the chain of survival and principles of DRABCD.
+ Detail how to question patients requiring first aid.
+ Describe the process for completing body checks on patients requiring first aid.
+ Describe the handover and referral of first aid patients to appropriate care.

how you may be assessed

underpinning knowledge

A number of oral or written questions may be asked relating to basic principles of first aid, the chain of survival, DRABCD, questioning patients, body checks and handover or referral of patients. Examples have been included at the end of the chapter.

practical demonstration

You may be required to demonstrate the principles of DRABCD on a patient. You may be asked to demonstrate how you would question a patient during first aid treatment. You may be required to perform body checks on a patient. You may be asked to demonstrate how you would handover or refer a patient to appropriate care after first aid and emergency care.

scenario

You may be required to demonstrate the principles of DRABCD, question a patient, perform body checks and prepare a patient for handover to appropriate care.

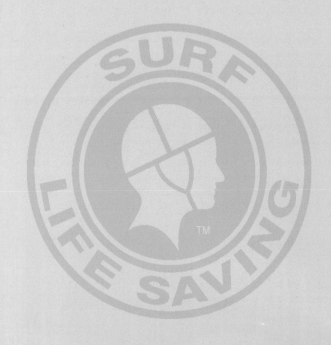

principles of management

The basic principles of management first aiders should be guided by are:

+ rapidly assess the situation (what has happened, how many patients there may be and their general condition)
+ check for danger to yourself, patient/s and bystanders
+ call for help
+ ensure your continued safety, as well as that of the patient/s and bystander/s
+ assess the response of each patient
+ the care of the unconscious patient has priority
+ stay with the patient, reassure them and continue to assess (it is vital that the first aider continually reassures the patient and explains everything that is being done).

Unless the condition is minor or there is great discomfort or danger, do not move the patient. Where there are risks from heat, cold, traffic, or other dangerous situations, immobilise fractures (if possible) before moving the patient (see Chapter 17). Treat the patient as if they had a spinal injury and immobilise and move properly if the event was not witnessed (see Chapter 21), after first establishing a clear airway. Airway management should always take precedence over spinal immobilisation.

An unconscious person who is breathing should be placed on their side to avoid choking and should be moved in this position.

When carrying a patient on a stretcher, ensure all movements are as smooth as possible and that the stretcher remains horizontal.

One of the most important, but often-neglected aspects of treatment, is reassuring the patient. Patients who have sustained an injury are often fearful of the results of their injury and unsure of what may happen.

signs and symptoms

Signs and symptoms are important tools that will help the first aider determine a person's condition. A sign is something that can be seen (objective evidence), such as bleeding, change in skin colour and limb deformity. A symptom is something a person can describe (subjective evidence), such as pain and nausea.

basic life support

The basics of life support are shown in the following flow chart. These basics relate to the principles of DRABCD detailed in the next section.

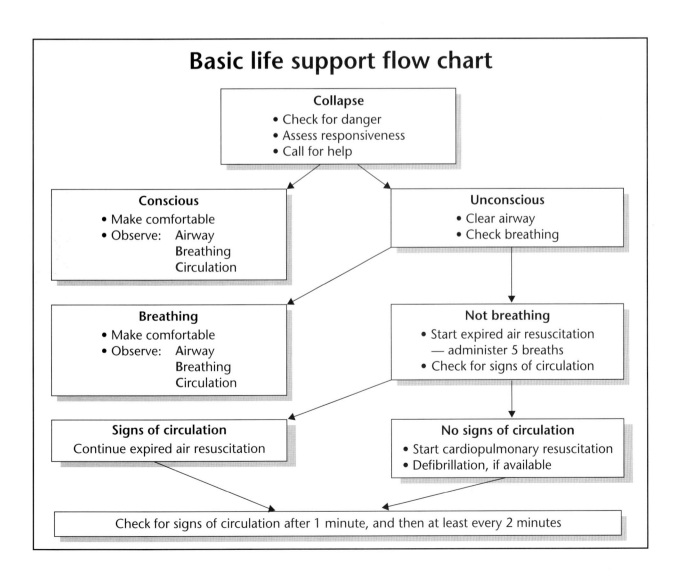

Basic life support flow chart

Collapse
- Check for danger
- Assess responsiveness
- Call for help

Conscious
- Make comfortable
- Observe: Airway
          Breathing
          Circulation

Unconscious
- Clear airway
- Check breathing

Breathing
- Make comfortable
- Observe: Airway
          Breathing
          Circulation

Not breathing
- Start expired air resuscitation — administer 5 breaths
- Check for signs of circulation

Signs of circulation
Continue expired air resuscitation

No signs of circulation
- Start cardiopulmonary resuscitation
- Defibrillation, if available

Check for signs of circulation after 1 minute, and then at least every 2 minutes

the chain of survival

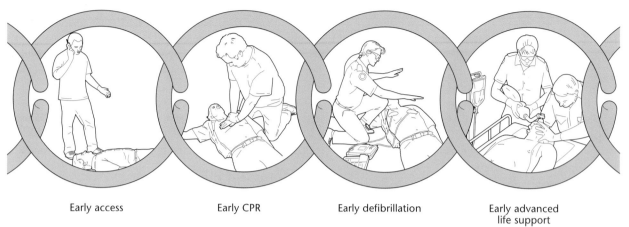

Early access   Early CPR   Early defibrillation   Early advanced
life support

The chain of survival

The assessment and management of a collapsed person is based on the idea of the 'chain of survival'. This involves:

✚ early access (contact emergency services: 'Call 000')
✚ early CPR (cardiopulmonary resuscitation; see Chapter 5)
✚ early defibrillation (see Chapter 24)
✚ early advanced life support.

For a patient to have the best chance of survival, first aiders must act quickly to assess the patient's condition, seek medical aid, and begin resuscitation.

Resuscitation is the preservation or restoration of life by establishing and maintaining a person's airway, breathing and circulation.

When calling for medical assistance, first aiders must consider a number of factors:

✚ the severity of the patient's condition
✚ availability of bystanders to call for help
✚ availability of ways and means (including modes of communication) to seek help.

There are no fixed rules for seeking assistance, as every scenario is different. However, some situations require more urgent medical assistance than others. A drowning patient, for example, will require oxygen immediately — getting oxygen into the patient's lungs via expired air resuscitation (EAR) is of paramount importance. A patient suffering a heart attack may require defibrillation, so it is important to call emergency services immediately, as specialised equipment and trained personnel may be essential for survival.

All patients who require resuscitation must be sent to hospital.

DRABCD

The principles of DRABCD apply to all first aid cases. These principles guide first aiders in their assessment and management of a patient.

| **Danger** |
| **Response** |
| **Airway** |
| **Breathing** |
| **Circulation** |
| **Defibrillation** |

danger

Assess the area for danger to yourself, the patient/s or bystander/s.

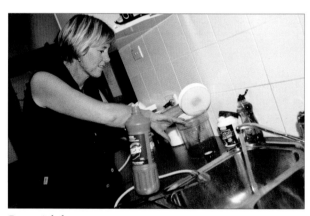

Potential dangers

Check the area around the site of the incident for items that may cause further injury to the patient or prevent you from helping them (e.g. broken glass, electricity cables).

Move the patient only if it is safe to do so and if the danger cannot be removed (e.g. removing a patient from a swimming pool).

If neither the patient nor the danger can be removed safely, seek expert assistance (e.g. electrical company, fire fighters, surf lifesavers). Remember that you cannot assist others if you add yourself to the casualty list by exposing yourself to danger.

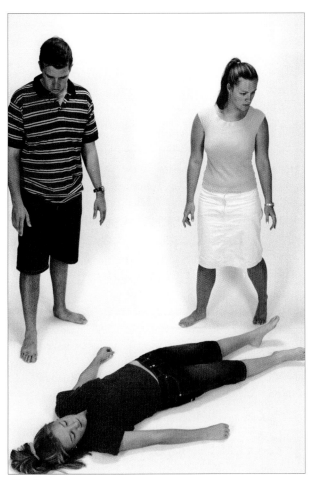

Check for danger

response

Assess the patient's level of consciousness by gently squeezing the patient's shoulders, taking care not to move the neck, and asking the patient to squeeze your hands or to open their eyes.

If there is no response to gentle squeezing or simple commands, the person must be regarded as unconscious, and assessment and care of the airway, breathing and circulation become a priority.

A conscious patient should be carefully assessed, made comfortable and managed according to the signs and symptoms exhibited.

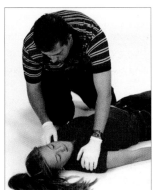 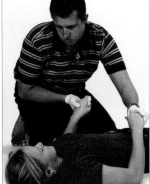

Check for response

airway

The key to successful resuscitation is a clear airway. Tilt the head backwards and lift the jaw using jaw support (see Chapter 4).

Look in the patient's mouth to see whether the tongue or foreign matter blocks the upper airway.

If the patient has *not* been rescued from the water or has *no* signs of vomit or fluid in or around the mouth, their airway and breathing can be assessed in the position found or on their back.

If the patient has been rescued from the water or there is obvious vomit and fluid in or around the mouth, roll them onto their side using the hip and shoulder roll.

 NOTE:
All unconscious persons and those recovering from a state of unconsciousness can be nursed on their side with careful attention given to the airway. The patient may be placed on either side of their body.

hip and shoulder roll

+ Place the patient's left arm outwards at right angles to the body, palm upwards, so that the radial pulse can be monitored.
+ Flex the patient's right hip to approximately 90 degrees by raising the knee and sliding the foot up towards the buttocks (acting as a lever when the patient is turned).
+ Place the patient's right arm across their chest and then, with your hands on the patient's shoulder and hip, gently roll the patient over onto their side.

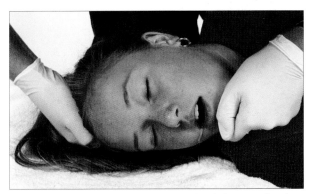

If there is obvious fluid or vomit around the mouth, place the patient on their side

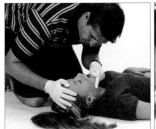 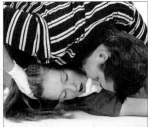

Checking the airway

clearing the airway

Keep the patient's head tilted back with the face turned slightly downward, if on their side. This position allows drainage of fluids and mucus from the mouth. Look in the patient's mouth to see whether the upper airway is blocked by the tongue or foreign material. Using the fingers, clear away any material such as vomitus, preferably wearing gloves (do not waste time waiting for them). Do not remove dentures unless they are loose and interfering with the patient's airway.

If there is no vomit or fluid around the patient's mouth, the airway can be cleared with the patient on their back.

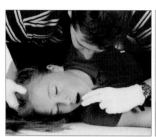 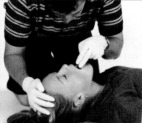

Clearing the airway

To open the airway tilt the patient's head backward, with the jaw held forward. The jaw may be held either at the chin (jaw support) or at the back of the jaw (see Chapter 4).

breathing

With the patient on their side or back, check for breathing using the principles of 'look, listen and feel'.

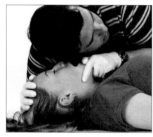 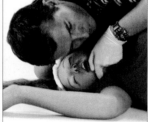

Look, listen and feel

+ *Look:* look down towards the chest and upper abdomen, checking for movement.
+ *Listen:* listen for sounds of air entering and leaving the lungs, with your ear about 5 cm from the patient's nose and mouth.
+ *Feel:* with your cheek over the patient's mouth and nose, feel for any movement of air from the patient's mouth or nose.

Usually, the decision on whether a patient is breathing is easy, but a brisk breeze or other ambient noise can cause problems when assessing the patient's breathing. If there is doubt about whether the patient is breathing, assume they are not, and start ventilation immediately (called expired air resuscitation, EAR; see Chapter 4).

Give 5 breaths in approximately 8–10 seconds, watching for the rise and fall of the patient's chest. Turn your head slightly to the side between breaths, to ensure a fresh breath of air is given to the patient each time and to listen/feel for air escaping from the lungs.

If breathing is present or returns, carefully place the patient in the lateral position and monitor the airway, breathing and circulation.

circulation

After completing 5 breaths, assess the patient's circulation, including their pulse, colour, temperature, breathing and any sign of movement. If there are no signs of circulation, start cardiopulmonary resuscitation (CPR; see Chapter 5).

defibrillation

If the signs and symptoms of circulation are absent (cardiac arrest) and a defibrillation (SAED/AED) unit and trained operator are available, defibrillation should be started as soon as possible (see Chapter 24). CPR should be continued until the unit is ready and should resume if defibrillation is unsuccessful (see Chapter 5).

patient questioning

In addition to observing the scene and the general appearance of the patient, it is important to question the patient to determine what happened and what treatment is needed. After introducing yourself, simple questioning will help you determine the general condition of the patient and whether there are any relevant current or past medical conditions that may influence treatment. It may also be appropriate to question a parent, guardian, companions or bystanders who may have witnessed the incident and may know more about the circumstances of events than the patient. Patient questions appear in Appendix 4.

body checks

Body checks are an important secondary assessment procedure that should be undertaken after life-threatening problems have been managed and medical aid is on the way. First aiders should look for any bleeding and other injuries, such as burns and fractures, as well as tenderness, swelling, wounds or deformity.

This secondary assessment should reveal any further problems to determine continuing treatment for the patient. Look, listen, feel and smell as the patient is being examined.

+ *Look*: for bleeding, skin colour and condition, and deformity.
+ *Listen*: for patient responses or sounds.
+ *Feel*: (very gently) for deformity, texture, swelling, or temperature.
+ *Smell*: the patient's breath and other odours to form an impression of other problems the patient may have.

body checks

A full body check should be carried out in the following order:

1. Neck, up over head and down across face

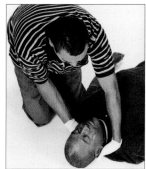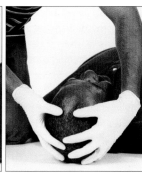

➕ Feel the spine gently (without moving the patient) for abnormalities of neck or swelling of soft tissue of throat

➕ Check scalp for lacerations, swelling or indentations indicating fractures

➕ Check ears for discharge of blood or clear fluid

➕ Check eyes for redness, irritation and foreign bodies; check pupils for size and ability to fix and follow

➕ Check nose for damage and bleeding

➕ Check mouth for loose teeth or bleeding

➕ Check skin colour for indications of lack of oxygen

2. Shoulders and front of chest, abdomen and pelvis including ribs

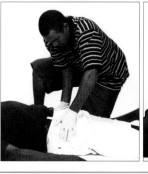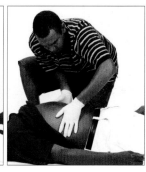

➕ Check skin for lacerations, penetrating wounds and colour

➕ Check that there is equal movement of chest wall during breathing

➕ Check pelvis for abnormal movement and fracture, and pain on movement and handling

➕ Note that an erection (in males) may be a sign of a spinal injury

3. Front and back of upper limbs

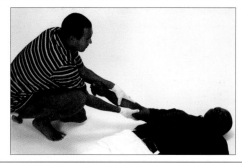

➕ Check shoulder joint for dislocation and fracture of bones

➕ Check skin for needle marks

➕ Check movement of joints and fingers for injury and pain on movement and handling

4. Front and back of lower limbs

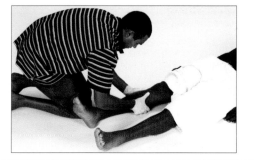

➕ Check knee and ankle joints and bones for injury and fractures

➕ Check skin for cuts and abrasions

➕ Determine whether there is pain on movement and handling

5. Back

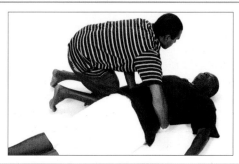

➕ Abnormal spinal appearance may indicate spinal injury

➕ Check skin for lacerations

handover

If an ambulance has been called, first aiders should stay with the patient, reassure them and continue to monitor them until the patient can be handed over to paramedics.

First aiders should introduce themselves and the patient to the paramedic and detail:

+ the events leading up to the incident
+ what happened to the patient
+ the patient's vital signs and times assessed
+ any injuries the patient has sustained
+ all treatment provided by the first aider.

All patients treated by a first aider should be referred to appropriate medical care for continuing or follow-up treatment. This includes referral to a health care professional.

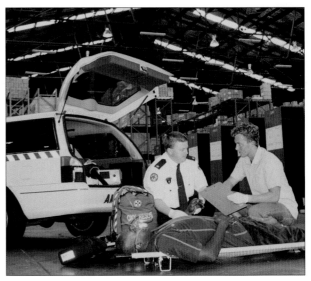

Handover to a paramedic

revision

1. What is the definition of a sign?

    _____

2. What is the definition of a symptom?

    _____

3. What are the four links in the 'chain of survival'?

    a) _____   b) _____

    c) _____   d) _____

4. For whom is it appropriate to assess breathing in the lateral position?
    a) All casualties should be assessed in the lateral position.
    b) Casualties who have obvious fluid or vomit around their mouth.
    c) Casualties who have been lifted from the water.
    d) Both b and c.

5. If a person has been assessed as not breathing, what should you do?
    a) Start cardiopulmonary resuscitation.   b) Check for signs of circulation.
    c) Deliver 5 breaths and check for signs of circulation.   d) b, then a.

6. If a person is not breathing and has no signs of circulation, what it the most appropriate thing to do?
    a) Start cardiopulmonary resuscitation and check for signs of circulation after 1 minute, and then at least every 2 minutes.
    b) Continue expired air resuscitation and check for signs of circulation after one minute.
    c) Defibrillation.
    d) a and c, if available.

7. When conducting a body check, what is the correct order? Fill in the correct number for each step below.

    ___ Shoulders and front of chest, abdomen and pelvis including ribs

    ___ Back

    ___ Front and back of upper limbs

    ___ Neck, up over head and down across face

    ___ Front and back of lower limbs

8. When handing a patient over to a paramedic, what information about the patient should you tell the paramedic?

    a) _____

    b) _____

    c) _____

    d) _____

    e) _____

Answers appear in Appendix 8.

expired air resuscitation (EAR)

learning outcomes

Perform expired air resuscitation (EAR) using approved methods and approaches.

+ Describe the breathing (respiration) process.
+ Detail the various methods of performing EAR in first aid and emergency care.
+ Detail the complications that may occur during EAR and how to rectify them.
+ Demonstrate the resuscitation of adults, children and infants using an appropriate simulation device.
+ Detail the oxygen-assisted resuscitation process.
+ Describe the precautions that must be observed during resuscitation.

how you may be assessed

underpinning knowledge

A number of written or oral questions may be asked relating to the breathing process, methods of EAR, identifying and rectifying complications with patients receiving EAR, resuscitation of infants and children, oxygen-assisted resuscitation and precautions. Examples have been included at the end of the chapter.

practical demonstration

You may be asked to show various methods of EAR on adults, children and infants. You may be required to demonstrate how you would rectify any complications that may arise during EAR on a patient. You may be required to demonstrate oxygen-assisted resuscitation.

scenario

You may be required to perform EAR on a simulation device with or without the assistance of oxygen.

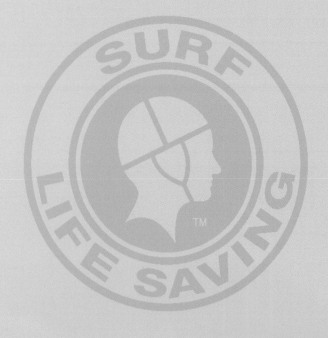

the chain of survival

The assessment and management of a collapsed person is based on the idea of the 'chain of survival' (see Chapter 3). This involves:

+ early access (contact emergency services: Call 000; see Chapter 3)
+ early cardiopulmonary resuscitation (CPR; see Chapter 5)
+ early defibrillation (see Chapter 24)
+ early advanced life support.

the breathing process

Breathing (respiration) is an involuntary reflex controlled by the breathing control centre in the brainstem. It is the act of moving air into and out of the lungs. During inspiration (inhalation), oxygen diffuses into the capillaries surrounding the alveoli in the lungs and carbon dioxide diffuses into the alveoli. Air from the lungs is then expelled during expiration (exhalation).

This process provides enough oxygen to meet the requirements of body tissues and organs. If breathing stops, tissues rapidly become hypoxic (low concentration of oxygen), leading to progressive brain damage and death if breathing is not re-established within 3–5 minutes. Prompt expired air resuscitation (EAR) can supply the body with sufficient oxygen until the patient begins to breathe again or until medical help arrives.

assessment prior to starting EAR

Having checked for 'Danger' and 'Response', the patient's breathing needs to be assessed.

+ If the patient has *not* been rescued from water or has *no* signs of vomit or fluid in or around the mouth, their airway and breathing can be assessed in the position they are found.
+ If the patient has been rescued from water, roll the patient onto their side for assessment.

To assess whether an unconscious person is breathing or not, you should:

+ *look:* look at the chest and upper abdomen, checking for movement
+ *listen:* listen for sounds of air entering and leaving the lungs, with your ear about 5 cm from the patient's nose and mouth
+ *feel:* with your cheek over the patient's mouth and nose, feel for any movement of air.

Environmental conditions (wind, noise) may make assessment difficult. If there is doubt about whether the patient is breathing, assume they are not. Carefully roll them onto their back (using a hip and shoulder roll if they are not already on their back), ensure the airway is open (see below), and start EAR immediately.

methods of EAR

For simplicity, this manual describes EAR from the patient's right side, as most right-handed first aiders feel more comfortable on that side. In reality, first aiders may perform resuscitation from either side, and it is important to practise so that you are proficient at giving EAR from either side.

The three methods of EAR are:

+ *mouth-to-mask resuscitation:* this is the preferred method to prevent infection and for first aider 'comfort' – some patients may vomit during CPR and EAR; first aiders should consider having pocket masks at home, at work or in the car
+ *mouth-to-mouth resuscitation*
+ *mouth-to-nose resuscitation.*

Each method is effective, provided that the patient's airway is clear, an effective seal is obtained and the first aider uses the correct force and rate of inflation.

	NOTE:	
	Rates of EAR	
	Adult patient	15 breaths per minute
	Child or infant patient	20 breaths per minute

Although the preferred position for resuscitation is with the patient on their back, it is possible for resuscitation to be performed in different positions. For example, in a car accident it may be impossible or unwise to remove the patient from the car, so EAR may be delivered with the patient in a sitting position.

mouth-to-mask resuscitation

This is the recommended form of respiratory resuscitation, and is a simple variation on the jaw thrust or jaw support method of holding the airway open. The general rules are the same as those described below for mouth-to-mouth resuscitation.

Backward head tilt is essential, except when a neck injury is suspected or the patient is an infant. The patient's jaw is held forward by the jaw thrust method and the first aider's thumbs (and index fingers, if necessary) are used to secure a firm seal between the mask and the patient's face. For this procedure, the first aider is usually positioned behind the head of the patient.

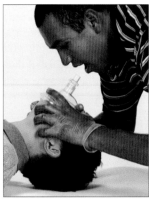
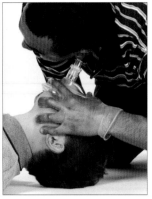

Mouth-to-mask resuscitation using the jaw thrust method

The first aider can also be positioned beside the patient and hold the mask down using the jaw support/pistol grip method, securing the bottom of the mask with the thumb holding the jaw and securing the top of the mask with the other hand.

applying pistol grip for mouth-to-mask resuscitation

+ Bend your middle finger and place it into the groove under the middle of the patient's chin.
+ Place your thumb over the bottom of the mask and over the patient's lower jaw.
+ Lay your index finger along the lower ridge of the jaw towards the ear.
+ Curl the middle, ring and small fingers in towards the palm of the hand.
+ Keep fingers clear of the soft tissues of the patient's throat and neck by keeping your elbow raised.
+ Lift the jaw upwards and outwards. This helps prevent the tongue from obstructing the airway.
+ Using your other hand, hold the top of the mask with your thumb and index finger.
+ The procedures for tilt, blow, look and look, listen and feel should be followed, as described below.

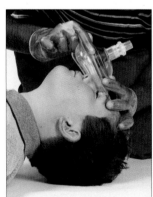
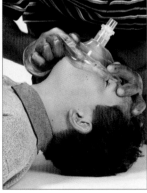

Mouth-to-mask resuscitation using the pistol grip method

mouth-to-mouth resuscitation

Once it is established that the patient is not breathing, the procedure is to:

+ turn the patient onto their back
+ tilt, blow, look
+ look, listen and feel.

tilt

+ Kneel beside the patient's head.
+ Place the palm of one hand on the patient's forehead.
+ Support the chin with the other hand and firmly, but gently, tilt the head backwards. This is referred to as 'head tilt'.
+ Support the chin by wrapping your index finger around the line of the patient's jaw, with the inside of your first knuckle in line with the point of the jaw.
+ Hold the little and ring fingers clear of the soft tissue of the neck.
+ Place the thumb along the front of the lower jaw between the lower lip and the point of the patient's chin.
+ Use the thumb to open the patient's mouth slightly. This is called 'jaw support'.

blow (inflation)

+ Take a deep breath, open your mouth as widely as possible and place it over the patient's slightly open mouth, sealing the nose with your cheek.
+ Blow gently to inflate the patient's lungs.

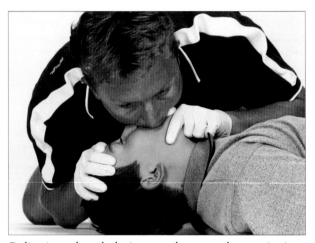

Delivering a breath during mouth-to-mouth resuscitation

look

Look for the rise of the patient's chest with each breath delivered. Blow until the patient's chest rises.

Possible causes of the chest not rising are:

+ an ineffective breath
+ obstruction in the airway (inadequate head tilt or jaw support, tongue blockage or foreign material obstruction)
+ insufficient air being blown into the lungs
+ inadequate air seal (air leak).

An air leak is indicated by:

+ air escaping around the mouth or nose.
+ failure of the chest to rise (as described above).

Sealing the patient's nose is necessary during mouth-to-mouth resuscitation, and this is best done with the first aider's cheek. Occasionally, air will continue to escape from the patient's nose. In such cases, it is necessary to pinch the nose, sealing the nostrils with your thumb and forefinger.

NOTE:
Take care to ensure that head tilt is maintained when sealing the nostrils with thumb and forefinger.

look, listen and feel (deflation)

+ After breathing into the patient, turn your head and place your ear about 5 cm from the patient's mouth to listen for and feel the air leaving the patient's mouth and nose.
+ Watch the patient's chest return to its original position.
+ Watch the upper abdomen and maintain head tilt to ensure that the stomach is not becoming swollen with air (distension).

NOTE:
The most common errors in resuscitation are loss of head tilt and over-inflation.

mouth-to-nose resuscitation

The mouth-to-nose resuscitation method may be used:

+ if the first aider prefers this method
+ in deep-water resuscitation (refer to SLSA Training Manual 32nd ed)
+ for resuscitating infants, when the first aider's mouth may not cover the infant's mouth and nose
+ if the patient's jaw is tightly clenched
+ in cases where severe facial injuries make it the preferable method.

The technique for mouth-to-nose resuscitation is similar to that used for mouth-to-mouth resuscitation, with some exceptions, as detailed below.

sealing the airway

+ Close the patient's mouth with the hand supporting the jaw.
+ Push the lips together with your thumb.

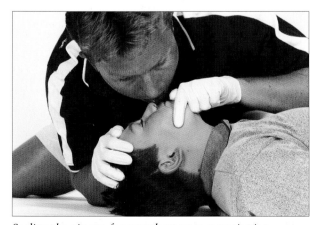

Sealing the airway for mouth-to-nose resuscitation

blow (inflation)

+ Take a breath and place your widely opened mouth over the patient's nose.
+ Take care that your mouth completely encloses the bridge of the patient's nose. Do not compress the soft part of the patient's nose.
+ Blow gently to inflate the patient's lungs.

look, listen and feel (deflation)

+ Lift your mouth from the patient's nose.
+ Using your thumb, peel down the patient's lower lip — there is no need to open the patient's mouth.
+ Look for the fall of the chest.
+ Listen and feel for air escaping from the nose and mouth.
+ Release the lower lip once exhalation is complete and push lips together before administering the next breath.

EAR for laryngectomy stoma

Patients who have had their larynx surgically removed breathe through a hole in their neck, called a stoma. Consider this possibility in patients wearing cravats or scarves around their neck, which act as an air filter.

Resuscitation is performed differently in a patient with a laryngectomy stoma, as EAR must be performed over the stoma, rather than the mouth or nose.

If the patient has been assessed as not breathing:

+ quickly turn them onto their back
+ place your open mouth over the stoma or tube
+ apply jaw support with the head in backward tilt, as this will make it easier for you to seal your mouth over the stoma
+ blow gently until the chest rises.

As in all resuscitation, the airway should be cleared before starting EAR. Check the stoma before you begin and, if the tube is blocked, use percussion to remove the blockage, as for routine removal of any foreign body obstruction.

Reasons for failure of the chest to rise during EAR include:

+ *blocked stoma*: remove blockage with percussion between shoulder blades
+ *inadequate seal over stoma*: backward head tilt may allow a better seal
+ *partial mouth/nose breathing*: the patient may have had a tracheostomy rather than a laryngectomy, allowing partial neck as well as mouth and nose breathing. In this case, seal the nose with your middle and index fingers and hold the mouth closed with your thumb under the chin. Breathe into the stoma and release your seal on the mouth and stoma after the chest rises to allow air to escape.

Complications during EAR
Foreign body airway obstruction (FBAO)

Suspected choking

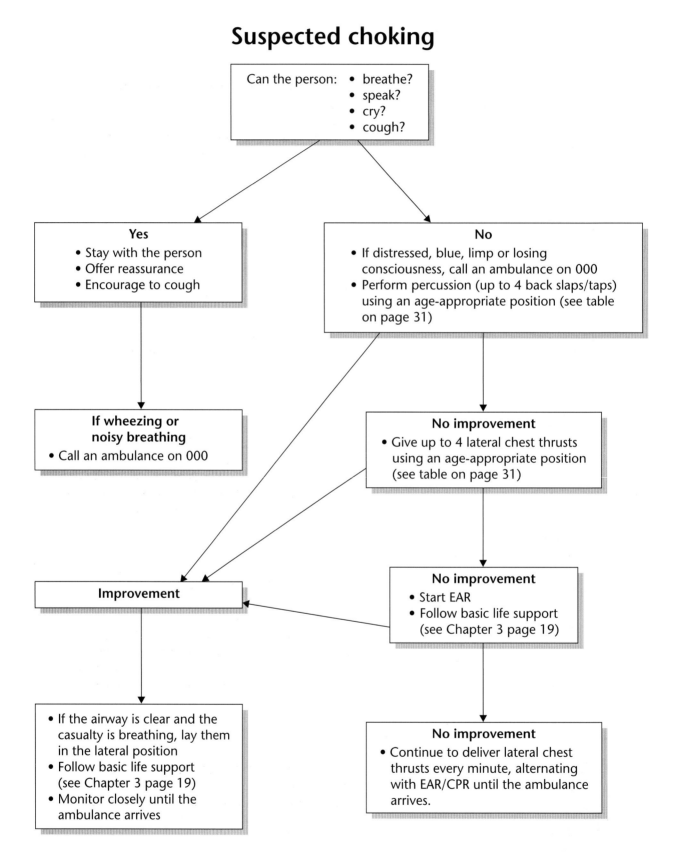

Can the person: • breathe?
                • speak?
                • cry?
                • cough?

Yes
• Stay with the person
• Offer reassurance
• Encourage to cough

No
• If distressed, blue, limp or losing consciousness, call an ambulance on 000
• Perform percussion (up to 4 back slaps/taps) using an age-appropriate position (see table on page 31)

If wheezing or noisy breathing
• Call an ambulance on 000

No improvement
• Give up to 4 lateral chest thrusts using an age-appropriate position (see table on page 31)

Improvement

No improvement
• Start EAR
• Follow basic life support (see Chapter 3 page 19)

• If the airway is clear and the casualty is breathing, lay them in the lateral position
• Follow basic life support (see Chapter 3 page 19)
• Monitor closely until the ambulance arrives

No improvement
• Continue to deliver lateral chest thrusts every minute, alternating with EAR/CPR until the ambulance arrives.

Based on foreign body airway obstruction material from the Australian Resuscitation Council
CPR = cardiopulmonary resuscitation; EAR = expired air resuscitation

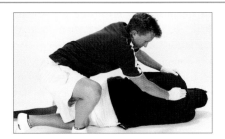

Percussion for adults:
+ Lay the person on their side
+ Deliver 3–4 slaps on the back between the shoulder blades

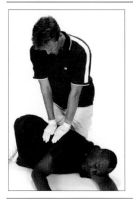

Lateral chest thrusts for adults:
+ Keep the patient lying on their side
+ Place one hand against the lower fold of the patient's armpit
+ Place your other hand beside the first and give 3–4 quick, forceful, downward thrusts, keeping your hands on the chest throughout

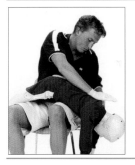

Percussion for children (1–8 yrs/up to 40kg):
+ Lay the child face down on your thigh, with their head hanging down
+ Deliver 3–4 gentle slaps on the back between the shoulder blades

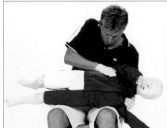

Lateral chest thrusts for children:
+ Lay the child on their side
+ Place one hand against the lower fold of the patient's armpit
+ Place your other hand beside the first and give 3–4 quick, downward thrusts, keeping your hands on the chest throughout

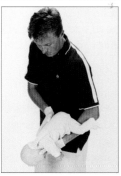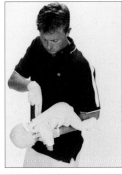

Percussion for infants (0–12 months):
+ Lay the infant on their stomach along your arm, supporting the chest with your hand, with the head extending beyond your hand and facing downward
+ If position alone is insufficient to remove the obstruction, deliver 3–4 two-finger taps on the infant's back between the shoulder blades

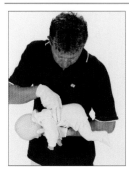

Lateral chest thrusts for infants:
+ Keep the infant face down
+ Place a hand on either side of the chest under the armpits
+ Give up to 4 quick, inward thrusts, keeping your hands on the chest throughout

partial airway obstruction

For a partially blocked airway, where an adult, child or infant is coughing and grabbing their throat:

+ encourage the patient to cough and observe their progress
+ reassure the patient.

If the obstruction is not removed by coughing, perform percussion and lateral chest thrusts, as appropriate for the person's age, as described below.

complete airway obstruction

If the patient's chest does not rise with inflation during EAR, check that:

+ the head is tilted back (except in young children and infants) and that the jaw is held forward correctly
+ there is no foreign material in the airway
+ the mouth/nose or mask seal is firm
+ enough air is being blown in.

If inflation is still not occurring after checking for the above, it is likely that there is foreign material in the back of the throat.

+ Place the patient in an age-appropriate position for percussion (see table on page 31).
+ Deliver 3–4 back slaps/taps (percussion).
+ Check airway.
+ If still obstructed, deliver 3–4 lateral chest thrusts in an age-appropriate manner (see table on page 31).
+ Clear and open the airway and re-check for signs of breathing.
+ If the airway is still blocked, try to blow the obstruction into the lungs by performing EAR. Gentle blows and puffs should be used for children and infants, respectively.
+ It may be necessary to perform CPR, after calling for an ambulance, if the blockage cannot be removed.

vomiting

Vomiting is the process in which muscular action makes the stomach eject its contents up into the oesophagus and out the mouth/nose. It is nearly always accompanied by a loud noise and does not occur if the patient is unconscious.

regurgitation

Regurgitation is the silent flow of stomach contents into the mouth and nose. This makes regurgitation dangerous, as it is difficult to detect.

Regurgitation does occur in an unconscious person, and is more likely when there is pressure on the abdomen (particularly when distended by air in the stomach). It is extremely common during resuscitation.

A person who regurgitates or vomits while lying face up is very likely to inhale some of the stomach contents into the lungs, which may lead to serious lung damage and infection.

Therefore, all unconscious, breathing people should be placed in the lateral position with their head tilted backward and the mouth pointing slightly downward, so that any stomach contents brought up drain on to the ground and are not inhaled (aspirated) back into the lungs. Vomiting and regurgitation, together with the loss of head tilt, are the most common problems likely to occur during resuscitation. It is vital to check and prevent these occurring — this cannot be stressed enough.

After clearing the airway, assess breathing and circulation. If breathing is not present, roll the patient onto their back and continue either EAR or CPR.

distension of the stomach

In cases of near drowning, the patient's stomach is often swollen at the time of rescue as they have swallowed great quantities of water and air.

This may be exacerbated by:

+ EAR performed with the airway partially blocked by the tongue or foreign material
+ the first aider blowing too hard (giving too much air)
+ poor or no head tilt (sending air down the oesophagus to the stomach).

A distended stomach can be recognised from a persistent and possibly increasing swelling in the upper part of the patient's abdomen.

NOTE:
A distended stomach leads to increased upward pressure on the lungs, making EAR more difficult. It also greatly increases the risk of regurgitation.

First aiders should not try to reduce the swelling of a patient's abdomen — leave the treatment of this condition to paramedics or hospital staff. Check that all procedures for correct EAR are being followed and that the airway is not blocked. Further stomach distension can be prevented by:

+ following the guidelines for maintaining a clear airway
+ watching for the rise and fall of the chest and the upper abdomen (the latter of which indicates air is entering the stomach)
+ blowing only until you see the chest rise
+ not blowing too quickly.

resuscitation of infants and children

An infant is a baby up to the age of 12 months, and a young child is defined as being aged between 12 months and 8 years. For infants and young children, the rules for resuscitation are a little different from those for an adult, although most basic principles are the same.

An infant's airway is more easily blocked than an adult's because:

+ the head is relatively large
+ the neck is relatively short
+ the tongue is large
+ the trachea (windpipe) is soft and easily compressed
+ the adenoids may be large.

Many infants and young children breathe through their nose, so it is important to clear the nose when checking the airway. Backward head tilt should not be used with infants as the soft tissue is easily compressed and may block the airway. It is generally not necessary in young children either, though children closer to the upper age limit (8 years) may require gentle head tilt to open the airway.

+ Keep the head in the neutral position (level), with the lower jaw supported at the point of the chin. If the neutral position does not provide a clear airway, it may be necessary to tilt the head back very slightly.
+ When performing EAR, place your mouth over the mask opening (or over the infant's nose and mouth, if no mask is available) and, with a slightly open mouth, puff in just enough air to cause the chest to rise. If you can't get an effective seal using a mask or with mouth-to-mouth, then use the mouth-to-nose method, as an infant's tongue may partially block the airway, causing the stomach to distend with the mouth-to-mouth method.
+ Using a mask, mouth-to-mouth and mouth-to-nose techniques are appropriate for young children.
+ The volume of air required for infants is very small. This procedure should be practised on infant manikins.
+ Infants and young children breathe faster than adults, so the rate of EAR is 1 small breath/puff every 3 seconds, or 20 breaths per minute.

Great care must be taken in judging the volume of air to be blown into the lungs of an infant or child, as blowing too much or too hard increases the risk of regurgitation and lung trauma. Blow *only* until the patient's chest is seen to rise.

In children older than 9 years of age, the rules and rate of breaths are the same as those for resuscitating adults.

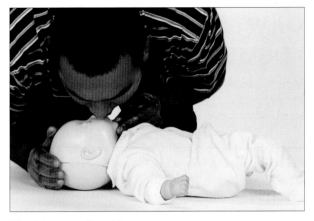

Head in neutral position

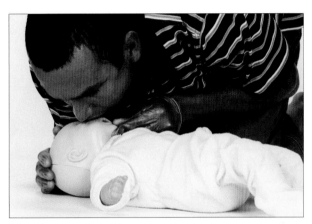

Head in neutral position using pistol grip

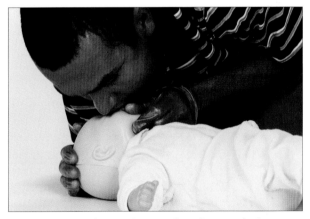

Place your mouth over the mouth and nose when resuscitating infants and give slow breaths/puffs until the chest rises

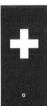

NOTE:
- The rate of EAR for infants and young children is 20 breaths per minute.
- Do not use backward head tilt in infants: minimal head tilt may be necessary in young children.
- Exercise great care when judging the volume of air to inflate the lungs of infants and young children. Puff or blow only until the chest rises.

oxygen-assisted resuscitation

Mouth-to-mask resuscitation can be more effective when oxygen is added (see Chapter 23). If oxygen equipment arrives, the trained operator may attach the tube to the special oxygen tubing connection on the mask. The tubing can also be placed through the main opening of the mask, where it is held in place by the EAR operator's fingers, or by the EAR operator's mouth as they breathe into the mask.

Practising this technique is essential.

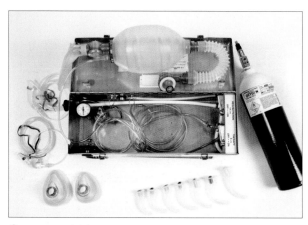

Oxygen equipment

precautions during resuscitation

First aiders should avoid direct contact with blood and other body substances of people being treated. It is strongly recommended that first aiders wear protective gloves and use a facial barrier for every case of resuscitation.

Several viruses and bacteria are present in human saliva. The following have been transmitted during mouth-to-mouth resuscitation:

+ tuberculosis
+ meningitis
+ cold sores (herpes simplex).

HIV and hepatitis have not been transmitted by resuscitation to date of publication, although transmission is theoretically possible. It is also possible for poisoning (e.g. insecticide poisoning) to occur during mouth-to-mouth resuscitation.

Apart from gloves, other barriers that may protect a first aider from the possibility of cross-infection include:

+ facemask
+ face shield.

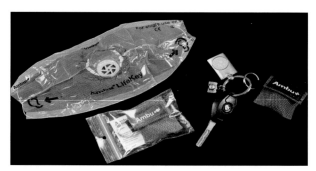

Face shield keyring

revision

1. Complete the following sentences about the breathing process.

    During .... (inhalation), oxygen diffuses into the .... surrounding the alveoli in the lungs and

    .... diffuses into the alveoli. Air from the .... is then expelled during expiration (..................).

2. When assessing a patient's breathing, what is meant by look, listen and feel?

    _____

    _____

    _____

    _____

3. How should you treat a partially blocked airway?

    _____

    _____

    _____

4. Which of the following statements about percussion is *not* true?
    a) Lay adults on their side and deliver 3–4 slaps on the back between the shoulder blades.
    b) Lay children face down on your thigh, with their head closest to your body and deliver 3–4 gentle slaps on the back between the shoulder blades.
    c) Lay infants on their stomach along your arm, supporting the chest with your hand, with the head extending beyond your hand and facing downwards and deliver 3–4 two-finger taps on the infant's back between the shoulder blades, if position alone is insufficient to remove the obstruction.

5. Why is regurgitation dangerous in the unconscious patient?

    _____

    _____

    _____

6. List five reasons why airway blockage is more common in infants than adults.

    a) _____

    b) _____

    c) _____

    d) _____

    e) _____

Answers appear in Appendix 8.

cardiopulmonary resuscitation (CPR)

learning outcomes

Perform cardiopulmonary resuscitation (CPR) using approved methods and approaches.

+ Detail when CPR is required.
+ Demonstrate the approach for CPR for adult patients.
+ Demonstrate the approach for CPR for infants and children.
+ Detail the modifications necessary when performing CPR on patients in the late stages of pregnancy.
+ Detail how long CPR should be performed.
+ Detail the management of patients after CPR.

how you may be assessed

underpinning knowledge

A number of written or oral questions may be asked relating to the need for CPR, the different applications of CPR on adults, children and infants, special considerations for performing CPR, how long CPR should be performed and patient management after CPR. Examples have been included at the end of the chapter.

practical demonstration

You may be asked to demonstrate CPR on adult, child and infant manikins. You may be required to demonstrate how you would rectify any complications that may arise during CPR on a patient. You may be required to demonstrate oxygen-assisted resuscitation.

scenario

You may be required to perform CPR on a casualty with or without the assistance of oxygen.

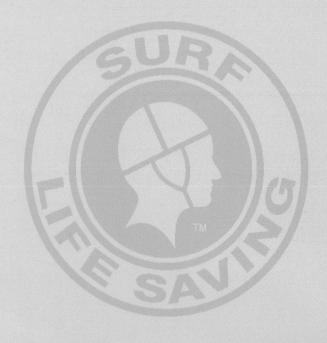

A person whose heart has stopped may be kept alive by a first aider who provides artificial ventilation of the lungs (expired air resuscitation — EAR) and artificial circulation of the blood (external cardiac compression — ECC). This combination of procedures is known as cardiopulmonary resuscitation (CPR).

ECC can provide circulation of blood after cardiac arrest by rhythmic compression of the heart between the breastbone (sternum) and the backbone (spine). The pumping is made more effective by a 'thoracic pump' effect, where the external compression increases the pressure inside the chest cavity, thereby increasing the effect of the compression of the heart.

Research has shown that the sooner CPR is begun, the greater the likelihood that the patient will survive.

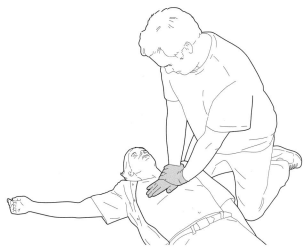

External cardiac compression

review of DRABCD

The principles of DRABCD apply to all resuscitations and guide your assessment and management of the patient.

> **D**anger — assess
>
> **R**esponse — check consciousness
>
> **A**irway — assess and clear
>
> **B**reathing — assess as present or absent, provide EAR if absent
>
> **C**irculation — assess as present or absent, provide CPR if absent
>
> **D**efibrillation — apply if available and necessary

CPR

CPR is required for patients who are unconscious, not breathing and have no signs of circulation.

The following five signs indicate a lack of circulation:

+ unconsciousness
+ absence of breathing
+ absence of movement
+ absence of the carotid pulse
+ skin colour that is pale or cyanosed (blue).

In some patients, a pulse is very difficult to find, especially in the elderly, in people removed from a cold environment and in overweight people.

finding and checking the pulse

+ Hold the head tilted backward with one hand on the patient's forehead. Place 2–3 relaxed fingers of the other hand on the patient's Adam's apple and slide them outwards (laterally) into the groove between the muscle of the neck (that runs from the bone behind the ear to the middle of the sternum) and the windpipe (trachea). In infants and young children, it may be easier to feel the brachial pulse, which is located on the inner (medial) side of the upper arm just above the elbow, or the apex heartbeat, which is just to the left of the lower half of the sternum. Remember to press gently at any site.
+ Feel for the pulse with the pads of the fingers (not the fingertips) for 5–10 seconds. Do not use your thumb.
+ Do not press too firmly or too lightly.
+ Do not feel both sides of the neck at the same time.

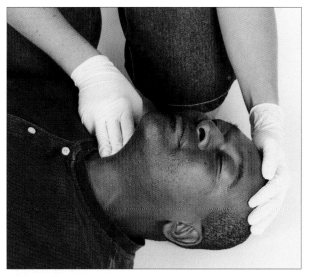

Feeling for the carotid pulse

If no pulse is detected, and no other signs of circulation are present, CPR should be started.

CPR for adults

hand position for first aiders

Kneel comfortably close to and alongside the chest of the patient, so that vertical pressure can be applied to the breastbone (sternum). This position will vary slightly for first aiders of different sizes and shapes. You can kneel on either side of the patient — procedures should be practised from both sides.

The patient's arm closest to you should be placed at right angles to the body, with the palm facing up. This allows easy access to the radial pulse for monitoring circulation.

Before starting CPR, it is important to correctly locate the site on the patient's chest to perform compressions.

➕ Feel along the bottom edge of the patient's lower ribs to where they join in the midline. The ribs meet at the bottom of the sternum and project downward towards the abdomen.

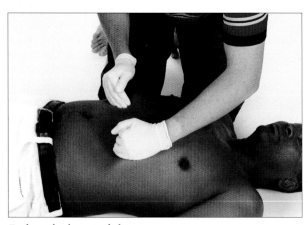

Feeling the lower rib line

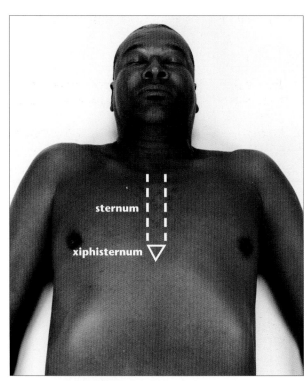

Location of sternum and xiphisternum

➕ Below where the ribs join in the midline is a small bone called the xiphoid process, or xiphisternum. This bone may be very difficult to locate in some people.

➕ Above the xiphisternum at the point where the ribs meet at the bottom of the sternum is a small notch. Mark this point with the middle finger of one hand. Place the index finger of the same hand next to it (towards the head). Place the heel of the other hand so it just touches this index finger. At all times the hand on the chest, referred to as the compressing hand, must remain above the xiphisternum, and on the lower half of the sternum.

➕ If the correct point is not found, compression may be too low on the chest. Not only will the heart be incompletely or insufficiently compressed, but the stomach may also be compressed causing regurgitation. It is also possible to damage organs in the upper abdomen. The callipering method may also be used to find correct hand position.

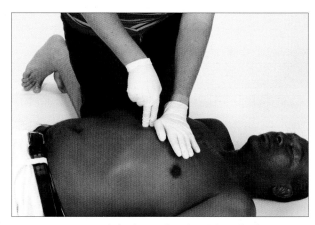

Correct position of the lower hand to identify the compression point

NOTE:
This is the preferred teaching and assessment method of SLSA. Other methods are recognised in Australian Resuscitation Council Policy Statements.

correct compression technique

➕ Once you have found the correct compression point, and placed the heel of the preferred hand on this point, relax and lift the fingers so that *all* pressure is applied to the patient's sternum and not to the ribs.

➕ Place the other hand securely on top of the first. To prevent the top hand slipping (and to avoid inaccurate compression), lock the fingers of the upper hand around the wrist of the lower hand. Alternatively, if one hand is placed on top of the other, the fingers may be interlocked. If your hands are not locked together, or fingers interlocked, there is greater risk that the force of compression will not be applied vertically through the correct point, making compression less effective or allowing the hands to slip on the chest, especially if they are wet.

+ Apply vertical pressure from your shoulder through the heel of the compressing hand, keeping the elbow of the compressing arm straight, and using the weight of your body as the compressing force. This takes less physical effort than trying to use the arm muscles, and is less tiring.
+ Compressions should be rhythmical, with equal time given to compression and relaxation. Extensive practise with a manikin is essential.
+ The sternum should be compressed one-third of the chest depth during CPR. In the average adult, this is between 4 and 5 cm.

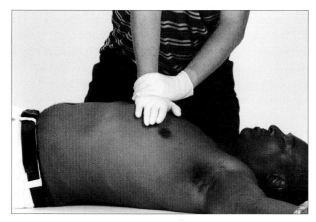

Vertical chest compression

co-ordination of EAR and ECC

In many situations, it may be necessary for one first aider to perform CPR alone and administer both EAR and ECC. However, when two first aiders are available to perform CPR, one should assume the role of the EAR operator and look after the patient's airway, while the other assumes the role of the ECC operator and looks after the circulation. Co-ordination is essential to ensure that the chest is not compressed while a breath is given (increasing the likelihood of air in the stomach).

Irrespective of whether one or two people are performing CPR, 2 breaths of expired air resuscitation are given for each 15 compressions. For one-person CPR, the 2 breaths should be given in approximately 4–5 seconds, and the 15 compressions given in 9–10 seconds, which allows for time to move between chest compression and delivering breaths.

oxygen-assisted resuscitation

Mouth-to-mask resuscitation can be more effective if additional oxygen can be delivered, as it increases the concentration of oxygen delivered to the patient (see Chapters 4 and 23). Oxygen can be supplied from an oxygen unit, if a unit and a qualified operator are available.

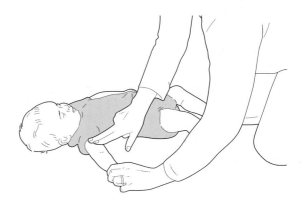

CPR for adults – 1 and 2 operators

+ Give 15 compressions and 2 breaths (one cycle) every 10–15 seconds, performing 4–6 cycles per minute.

CPR for infants and children

feeling the pulse

Assess the circulation of an infant (up to 12 months old) or child (1–8 years) as described for adults, except that the carotid pulse may not be as easy to detect in infants and young children. In this patient group, it is easier to feel the brachial pulse, located on the inner (medial) side of the arm in the elbow crease, or the apex beat of the heart, felt just to the left of the lower half of the sternum. Remember to press gently.

Feeling for the brachial pulse in an infant

compression

+ The compression point for children and infants is the lower part of the sternum, just as it is in adults, and is identified by the same method.
+ In infants, compression is performed using two fingers, to one-third of the chest depth (approximately 2 cm).

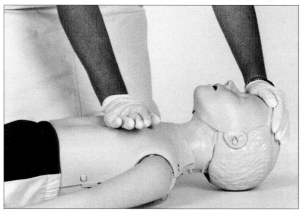

One-person CPR on a child

+ Compression can also be accomplished on infants by gripping the chest and gently squeezing your thumbs on the sternum at the usual location.
+ In young children (1–8 years of age), compression is performed using the heel of one hand to one-third of the chest depth (approximately 2–3 cm).

CPR for young children and infants – 1 and 2 operators

+ Give 5 compressions and 1 breath every 3 seconds as one cycle. Current information suggests that 5 compressions and 1 breath at or less than 3 seconds (one cycle) is more effective than 15 compressions to 2 breaths.
+ This means performing *at least* 20 cycles per minute with 100 compressions and 20 breaths.

Remember: Care must be taken not to compress the chest while a breath is given, as air will enter the stomach.

NOTE:
Two-person teams performing resuscitation, such as surf lifesavers and other similarly trained personnel, continue to use the existing team protocol of 5 compressions to 1 breath (see 32nd Ed SLSA Training Manual).

---

special considerations

pregnancy

Some modifications to CPR are required for women in the late stages of pregnancy.

The expanding uterus places upward pressure on the diaphragm, making EAR and chest compression more difficult. Also, compression may cause regurgitation and aspiration of the stomach contents.

It is not advisable to place a woman in the late stages of pregnancy flat on her back, as in this position the uterus may compress the major abdominal veins, impeding the return of deoxygenated blood to the heart. Wherever possible, she should be tilted to the left by placing a pillow or similar under the right hip, with the shoulders remaining flat and the left leg outwardly rotated and bent slightly (around 45 degrees). This will relieve pressure on the abdominal vessels while making EAR as easy as possible in the circumstances. If it is impossible to elevate the right hip, one rescuer or a bystander should gently hold the abdomen to the woman's left side. For this same reason, a pregnant woman should always be placed on her left side for recovery.

	ADULTS AND OLDER CHILDREN		**YOUNG CHILD**		**INFANT**	
Age	9 years and above		1–8 years		Up to 12 months	
Compress with	2 hands over lower half of sternum		Heel of 1 hand over lower half of sternum		2 fingers over lower half of sternum	
Depth of compression	One-third depth of chest (approx. 4–5 cm)		One-third depth of chest (approx. 2–3 cm)		One-third depth of chest (approx. 2 cm)	
Method	**1 person**	**2 person**	**1 person**	**2 person**	**1 person**	**2 person**
Compression: breaths	15:2	15:2	5:1	5:1	5:1	5:1
Timing per cycle (seconds)	10–15	10–15	3	3	3	3
Rate (compressions/minute)	60–100	60–100	100	100	100	100
Cycles per minute	4–6	4–6	20	20	20	20

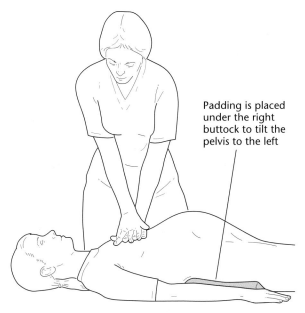

Padding is placed under the right buttock to tilt the pelvis to the left

The correct position for CPR on women in the late stages of pregnancy

management of the patient after CPR

✚ If you can see an improvement in colour and can feel a pulse, continue EAR until regular breathing starts.

✚ When breathing starts again, roll the patient into the lateral position and keep the airway open.

✚ Continually observe the patient's breathing, as it may stop, requiring you to undertake further resuscitation. If breathing is present, the pulse will also be present.

✚ Protect the patient from extremes of heat and cold — use blankets or shield the patient from the hot sun. Make sure that what you do does not interfere with your observation of the patient's airway and breathing.

✚ If the patient regains consciousness, make them comfortable and be gentle at all times.

✚ All patients who have received resuscitation *must* be referred to hospital.

 NOTE:
• Recovery may be only temporary. Continue to monitor the patient closely.
• Breathing may stop after early success with resuscitation — if this happens, EAR must be started again, along with the usual checks of the patient's circulation.
• The heart may also stop again — if this occurs, CPR must be started again, immediately.

how long should CPR continue?

CPR should continue until circulation and breathing return, or until:

✚ continuation poses a danger to the first aider
✚ someone takes over
✚ you cannot physically continue
✚ the patient is declared dead
✚ defibrillation starts.

 NOTE:
Don't give up — people have recovered after resuscitation attempts that have lasted over an hour.

revision

1. Which of the following statements about CPR is *not* true?
   a) ECC involves the rhythmic compression of the heart between the clavicle and the spine.
   b) ECC can provide circulation of blood after cardiac arrest.
   c) The sooner CPR is begun, the greater the likelihood that the patient will survive.
   d) CPR is combined EAR and ECC.

2. List the five signs to indicate a lack of circulation:

   a) _____   b) _____   c) _____

   d) _____   e) _____

3. What is the correct rate of compressions to breaths for adults?
   a) 5:1 for one operator, and 15:2 for 2 operators.
   b) 5:1 for both one and two operators.
   c) 15:2 for both one and two operators.

4. What is the correct rate of compressions to breaths for children and infants?
   a) 5:1 for one operator, and 15:2 for two operators.
   b) 5:1 for both one and two operators.
   c) 15:2 for both one and two operators.

5. Which of the following features of CPR are the same in adults, children and infants?
   a) Hand position.
   b) Compressions: breaths.
   c) Compression to one-third of depth of chest.
   d) a and c.

6. Why is CPR more difficult to perform on women who are in the late stages of pregnancy?

   _____

   _____

7. Why is it necessary to tilt women in the late stages of pregnancy slightly to the left during CPR?

   _____

   _____

8. CPR should continue until circulation and breathing return, or until:

   a) _____

   b) _____

   c) _____

   d) _____

   e) _____

9. Regarding care of the patient after CPR, which of the following is *not* true?
   a) Roll the patient into the lateral position when breathing starts and keep the airway open.
   b) Continually observe the patient's airway, breathing and circulation, as recovery may only be temporary and further resuscitation may be required.
   c) Protect the patient from extremes of heat and cold.
   d) Only complicated resuscitations need be referred to hospital.

Answers appear in Appendix 8.

bleeding

learning outcomes

Perform first aid to treat bleeding.

+ Demonstrate the standard treatment for a patient with external bleeding.
+ Describe the standard treatment for a patient with suspected internal bleeding.
+ Detail the management of bleeding under special circumstances.

how you may be assessed

underpinning knowledge

A number of oral or written questions may be asked relating to external bleeding, suspected internal bleeding and the management of bleeding during first aid and emergency care. Examples have been included at the end of the chapter.

practical demonstration

You may be asked to demonstrate how you would treat a patient with external bleeding. You may be asked to show how you would manage a patient with suspected internal bleeding. You may be asked to demonstrate how you would manage patients with bleeding under different circumstances.

scenario

You may be required to treat a patient with external and/or suspected internal bleeding detailing special circumstances relating to the bleeding.

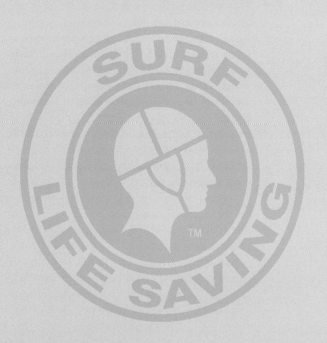

Most bleeding is superficial, easily recognised, relatively minor in quantity and easily stopped. Bleeding from an artery, however, is brisk and spurting, and needs immediate treatment.

At all times, avoid direct contact with the blood of the patient. Gloves should be worn, and changed after dealing with each patient. If gloves are not available, advise patients how to stop their own bleeding.

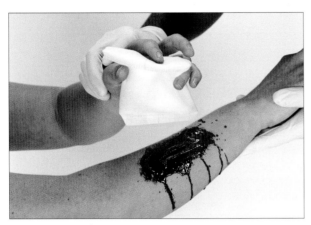

An open wound

Wherever possible, use sterile, prepacked disposable equipment, sterile dressings and clean bandages (see Chapter 11 for information on specific wounds and Chapter 12 for information on dressings and bandaging).

external bleeding

The *standard procedure* for treating a patient with serious bleeding is as follows.

+ Treat for shock (see Chapter 7).
+ Send others for medical help.
+ Application of direct pressure is the best way to control most bleeding. Use gloved fingers or the heel of the hand, using clean pads, towels or bandages whenever possible.
+ If the bleeding is from a limb, elevate it (after any fracture present has been immobilised).
+ Clean *around* minor wound sites with saline or warm soapy water, wiping away from the wound, gently removing any loose foreign material that may be present. Then, using fresh swabs, clean the wound area itself. Do not waste time trying to clean major bleeds.
+ Place a sterile dressing on the wound, maintaining direct pressure. If bleeding is heavy or a dressing is not available, grasp the sides of the wound and press them firmly together.
+ If bleeding persists, do not remove the dressing. Apply further pads and bandaging.
+ Administer oxygen therapy when available and qualified personnel are present.
+ Arterial tourniquets are *not* routinely recommended and should only be used as a 'last-resort' treatment in cases where major arteries have been severed (e.g. shark or crocodile attack or power-craft injuries) when

the usual conservative management is not effective and serious bleeding continues, placing the patient at risk of death from blood loss. *Send for urgent medical assistance, as tourniquets can cause irreparable damage if left on too long.*

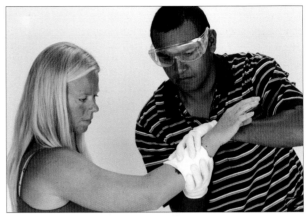

Apply clean, sterile pads

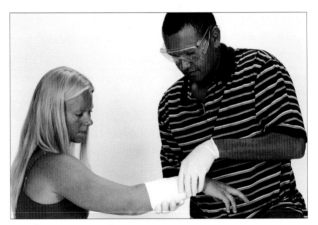

Bandage over a pad

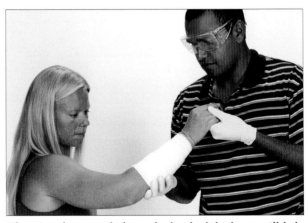

Elevating the wound above the level of the heart will help reduce bleeding

NOTE:
- Send for medical assistance, if required.
- Apply direct pressure.
- Raise the wound, if possible.
- Rest and reassure the patient.
- Administer oxygen therapy, if necessary and if equipment and suitably qualified personnel are present.

internal bleeding

Internal bleeding is usually very difficult for the first aider to recognise. Some internal bleeding has visible signs, such as bright red frothy blood coughed up from the lungs, vomiting blood or bleeding from an orifice (e.g. vagina, anus, ears). However, internal bleeding is often concealed. Signs of internal bleeding are usually those of shock (see Chapter 7) and include pale, cold, sweaty skin, shortness of breath, fast pulse and an altered state of consciousness.

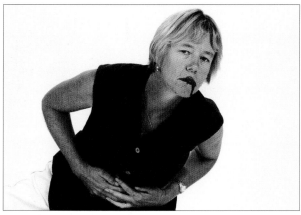

Bleeding from the mouth may indicate internal bleeding

signs

+ Swelling, limb deformity, redness or bruising associated with blood loss from a fracture
+ Increased pulse rate
+ A weak or thready pulse
+ Sweating
+ Pale skin
+ Bleeding from an orifice
+ Abdominal swelling — indicating major bleeding into the abdomen
+ Guarding of the area — patient lies still as movement causes pain, they may hold or clutch the affected area
+ Racoon eyes — bruising around the eyes (possibly indicating severe head trauma [fracture] to the base of the skull)

symptoms

+ Nausea
+ Abdominal pain
+ Feeling faint

treatment

+ Arrange urgent medical transport.
+ Rest the patient and reassure frequently.
+ Monitor airway, breathing and circulation (ABC).
+ Lay the patient down with legs slightly raised, if appropriate. Do not raise the legs if a head injury is suspected, and bend the knees if an abdominal injury is suspected.
+ Do not give the patient anything by mouth.
+ Oxygen should be administered, if a unit is available and qualified personnel present.

special circumstances

bleeding from the head

Bleeding from the head arising from small lacerations or cuts to the scalp often looks worse than it really is because the face and scalp have an abundant blood supply, and rupturing any of these superficial vessels causes profuse bleeding. Stem the bleeding by compressing around the wound and holding for 5 minutes, if the accident was not associated with any impact to the head.

If the bleeding was associated with an impact to the head, medical assistance is required. Even if there is no obvious damage to the skull, such as a depression at the site of injury, it is possible that the person may have sustained a skull fracture or damage to the brain — concussion, bruising (contusion) and bleeding into or around the brain (haemorrhage). Symptoms of head injuries include loss of consciousness (however transient), headache, vomiting, seizures, blurred vision, slurred speech, drowsiness and not feeling quite right. These symptoms generally emerge within 24 hours of the injury, though occasionally over longer periods.

When a cut is believed to have penetrated the skull, an object is embedded in the skull, or there is evidence of skull fracture — such as sunken, deformed areas, visible bone fragments or the brain is exposed — immediate medical assistance should be sought. These conditions are known as open head injuries and can be life-threatening. Monitor the symptoms of the head injury and observe the patient for signs of shock (see Chapter 7).

treatment

+ Send others for urgent medical help.
+ Reassure the patient and keep them still.
+ Do not attempt to move a person with suspected neck or spinal cord injury unless absolutely necessary.
+ Do not touch the site of injury.
+ Do not try and stop any bleeding or clear fluid draining from the ears.
+ Do not give the patient anything by mouth (especially aspirin, which promotes bleeding).

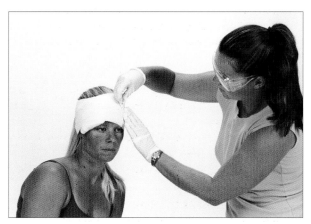

Applying a bandage to the head

bleeding from the ear

Bleeding or clear fluid from the ear may indicate a fractured skull or ruptured eardrum and should always be treated as a serious condition.

treatment

✚ If the patient is conscious, place them in a comfortable position with their head inclined to the injured side to allow the fluid to drain.

✚ If the patient is unconscious, place them on their side, injured side down, and manage their airway, breathing and circulation.

✚ Hold a loose dressing over the ear to absorb the fluid, but don't plug or attempt to block the ear.

✚ Seek urgent medical advice.

✚ Place the dressing or pad in a plastic bag and send with the patient for hospital analysis.

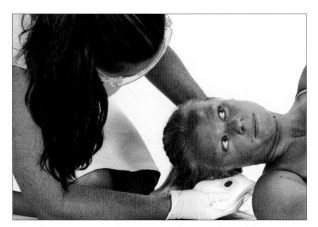

Lay the patient on their side with a sterile pad between the ear and the ground to absorb the blood/fluid

bleeding from the nose

The treatment for any nosebleed not associated with other injury is as follows.

✚ Sit the patient with their head bent forward. Squeeze the soft part of the nostrils just below the bone between the thumb and forefinger for up to 10 minutes.

✚ During this time, gently and slowly release pressure on the nostrils. Tell the patient to breathe through their mouth and not to blow or sniff through their nose. You may also apply a wet cloth to the back of the neck.

✚ Slowly release the compression after 10 minutes, reminding the patient not to blow or sniff through the nose.

✚ If bleeding does not stop within 10 minutes, or starts again after the initial bleeding stops, seek medical help.

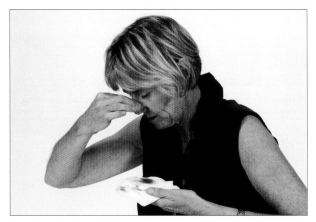

Apply pressure to the soft tissue of the nose for up to 10 minutes to stem bleeding

For nose bleeding following injury to the head, the initial treatment is much the same, taking care the nose is pressed only gently. A patient with a bleeding nose resulting from injury should always be advised to seek medical help.

It is advisable to check if the patient has any condition that may make them more prone to bleeding.

revision

1. Complete the following sentence about wound treatment when there is serious bleeding.

   Remember to apply .... pressure, raise the .... if possible, rest and .... the patient

   and .... for medical help.

2. What should you do if bleeding persists after bandaging?
   a) Remove and re-bandage.
   b) Apply further pads and bandaging.
   c) Apply pressure.

3. When is it appropriate to use arterial tourniquets?
   a) Never.
   b) For most major arterial bleeds.
   c) Only as a last resort when the patient is likely to die from blood loss without intervention.

4. List the possible symptoms of internal bleeding.

   a) _____   b) _____   c) _____

5. What are some signs of an open head injury?

   a) _____

   b) _____

   c) _____

6. Complete the following sentences about how to deal with bleeding from the nose.

   Sit the patient with their head bent .... Squeeze the .... part of the nostrils just below the

   .... between the thumb and forefinger for up to .... minutes.

Answers appear in Appendix 8.

shock

learning outcomes

Perform first aid to manage shock.

+ Detail the causes of shock.
+ Describe the signs and symptoms of shock.
+ Demonstrate the standard treatment for a patient with shock.

how you may be assessed

underpinning knowledge

A number of written or oral questions may be asked relating to the causes, signs, symptoms of and treatment for shock. Examples have been included at the end of the chapter.

practical demonstration

You may be asked to demonstrate how you would identify a patient suffering from shock. You may be asked to demonstrate how you would treat a patient suffering from shock.

scenario

You may be required to treat one or more patients suffering from shock.

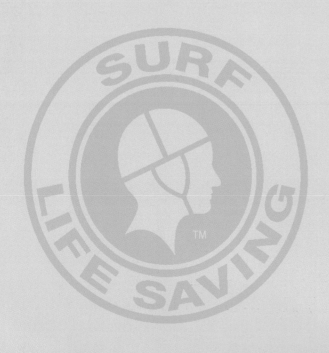

Shock is a medical term used to describe the loss of effective circulation — oxygen supply to the tissues suddenly becomes inadequate to meet the body's needs, especially to vital organs, such as the brain, lungs and heart.

Urgent medical advice is necessary in all cases of shock — untreated shock can kill.

causes of shock

Shock can be caused by any condition, though is commonly associated with:

+ blood loss
+ fluid loss
+ burns (see Chapter 16)
+ sweating and dehydration (heat stroke, see Chapter 16)
+ severe diarrhoea and vomiting
+ cardiac emergencies (see Chapter 9)
+ severe brain or spinal cord injury
+ severe infections
+ allergic reactions
+ major or multiple fractures
+ major trauma.

NOTE:
Witnessing severe traumatic events does not cause true shock (circulatory collapse), but the resulting condition requires specialised medical attention.

TYPE OF SHOCK	CAUSE
Hypovolaemic shock	Inadequate blood volume (loss of one fifth or more of the normal blood volume), due to blood loss or excessive loss of body fluids
Cardiogenic shock	Damage to the heart, so that it is unable to pump enough blood to meet the nutritional needs of the tissues
Neurogenic shock	Damage to the brain or spinal cord
Anaphylactic shock	Severe allergic reaction
Septic shock	Systemic infection, leading to dilation of blood vessels and, therefore, reduced blood pressure and blood flow to the tissues

signs

Signs of shock appear within the first hour of an injury/accident.

+ Reduced level of consciousness
+ Confusion
+ Vomiting
+ Rapid breathing or 'air hunger'
+ Pale, cold, clammy skin (lips and fingernails may appear blue)
+ Enlarged (dilated) pupils
+ Rapid, weak pulse
+ Inability to palpate radial pulse (suggesting low blood pressure)

symptoms

+ Faintness or dizziness
+ Trembling or weakness in the arms and legs
+ Nausea
+ Restlessness, anxiety

treatment

Try to anticipate shock in patients with severe injuries or infection. Early intervention and appropriate care may prevent shock from developing and will save lives.

+ Seek medical help urgently.
+ Lay the person on their back in a horizontal position (to improve circulation). Do not elevate the head.

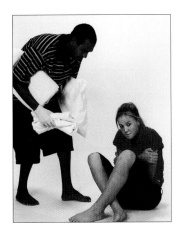

Assisting a patient in shock

+ If head injury is not suspected, raise the patient's legs, keeping the head level with the heart.

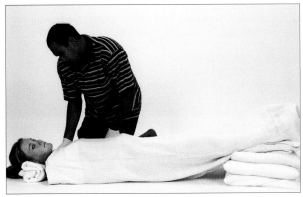

If a head injury is not suspected, raise the legs

- Turn the unconscious patient on their side and monitor their airway, breathing and circulation.
- Loosen any tight clothing.
- Protect the patient from extremes of temperature.
- Moisten the patient's lips, but do not give drinks or food.

- Administer oxygen therapy, if equipment and suitably qualified personnel are present.
- Monitor the patient closely, as they may deteriorate rapidly.
- If the patient does deteriorate, administer EAR and CPR, as appropriate.

revision

1. Which of the following are *not* causes of shock?
   a) Blood loss.
   b) Minor infections.
   c) Burns.
   d) Severe diarrhoea and vomiting.

2. What is the cause of hypovolaemic shock?

   _____

   _____

3. What is the cause of septic shock?

   _____

   _____

4. What are the symptoms of shock?

   a) _____

   b) _____

   c) _____

   d) _____

5. What is the correct position in which to place a conscious person in shock until medical help arrives?

   _____

   _____

6. How would you modify this position if you suspected the person had sustained a head injury?

   _____

   _____

Answers appear in Appendix 8.

respiratory emergencies

learning outcomes

Perform first aid to manage respiratory emergencies.

- Describe the causes of respiratory distress.
- Detail appropriate treatment for a patient who has drowned or nearly drowned.
- Detail the signs of and treatment for a patient with laryngeal spasm.
- Detail the signs and symptoms of and treatment for a patient who is hyperventilating.
- Detail the causes, signs and symptoms of and treatment for a patient suffering from an asthma attack.
- Demonstrate the standard treatment for a patient who has suffocated.
- Demonstrate the standard treatment for a patient suffering from smoke or gas inhalation.
- Detail the signs and symptoms of and treatment for a patient suffering an allergic reaction.
- Detail the signs and symptoms of and treatment for a patient with chest injuries.
- Detail the signs and symptoms of and treatment for a patient who has been winded.

how you may be assessed

underpinning knowledge

A number of written or oral questions may be asked relating to the cause of respiratory distress, drowning or near drowning, laryngeal spasm, hyperventilation, asthma, suffocation, smoke or gas inhalation, allergic reactions, chest injuries and winding. Examples have been included at the end of the chapter.

practical demonstration

You may be asked to demonstrate how you would treat a patient who has drowned or nearly drowned. You may be asked to demonstrate how you would recognise and treat a patient with laryngeal spasm. You may be asked to demonstrate how you would treat a patient who is hyperventilating. You may be asked to demonstrate how you would treat a patient suffering from an asthma attack. You may be asked to demonstrate how you would treat a patient who has suffocated. You may be asked to demonstrate how you would treat a patient suffering from smoke or gas inhalation. You may be asked to show how you would treat a patient with an allergic reaction. You may be asked to show how you would treat a patient with chest injuries. You may be asked to demonstrate how you would treat a patient who has been winded.

scenario

You may be required to treat one or more patients suffering from a respiratory emergency.

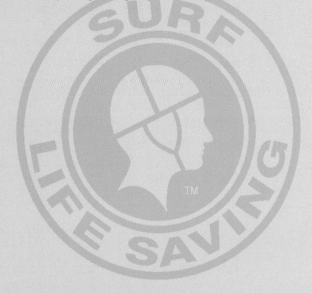

identifying respiratory distress

Many problems may affect a patient's ability to breathe, ranging from chronic conditions, such as asthma and bronchitis, to acute presentations where someone may have inhaled toxic fumes or developed an obstruction in their airway. The patient in respiratory distress requires continuous monitoring and immediate transport to hospital.

Determining respiratory distress involves assessing six criteria, as shown in the table below.

- If the patient is not breathing, start EAR (see Chapter 4) delivering 5 breaths before checking for the carotid pulse.
- If there is no pulse, start CPR (see Chapter 5) and continue until the patient recovers or medical help arrives.
- Administer oxygen, if a unit is available and a qualified operator is present.

 NOTE:
After retrieval, assessment in the lateral position and early oxygenation are the cornerstones of treatment.

drowning/ near drowning

Drowning is death by suffocation from immersion in water or other liquid, whether or not the medium has entered the lungs.

Near-drowning is the term used when a patient survives for more than 24 hours.

treatment

- Follow DRABCD (see Chapter 3).
- Remove the patient from the water/liquid without placing yourself at risk.
- Have someone call an ambulance immediately.
- Open and clear the airway of the unconscious patient.
- Assess respiratory function with the patient on their side, in case of vomiting or regurgitation.

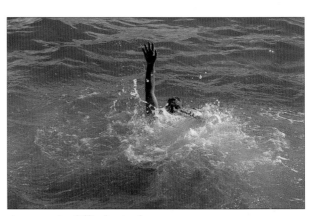

A person in difficulty in the water

laryngeal spasm

Laryngeal spasms are observed in some inflammatory or infectious conditions, allergic reactions and, occasionally, in cases of drowning. Laryngeal spasms restrict or

CRITERIA	NORMAL	ABNORMAL
1. Respiratory rate	*Adult:* 12–16 breaths per minute *Child:* 20 breaths per minute	*Adult:* <10 breaths per minute or >20 breaths per minute *Child:* <15 breaths per minute, or >25 breaths per minute
2. Respiratory rhythm (observe patient's chest)	Rise and fall of chest is regular and even	Rise and fall of chest is irregular and uneven
3. Respiratory effort (observe patient's chest and neck)	Usually only a small amount of chest movement during quiet respiration	Marked chest movement Use of accessory muscles to assist breathing (neck, abdomen, ribs)
4. Appearance	Calm and quiet	Anxious and distressed May be fighting for air or completely exhausted
5. Ability to speak	Clear flowing sentences	Short sentences or single words
6. Noises	No audible respiratory noises	Cough, stridor, inspiratory/expiratory wheeze or wet gurgling noises In severe episodes, the patient may make no noise

prevent air entering the lungs and, in severe cases, cause respiratory failure and death. Urgent medical attention is required and patients may require intubation. EAR is virtually impossible in these patients, due to restricted airflow, and only stomach distension occurs.

signs

+ Strangled voice sound
+ Inspiratory and expiratory loud wheezing (stridor)
+ Extreme difficulty breathing with the use of accessory breathing muscles (neck muscles and intercostal muscles in between the ribs can be seen dragging in)
+ Respiratory failure in severe cases

treatment

+ Immediately send someone to call for an ambulance.
+ Reassure and encourage the patient to relax and breathe deeply.
+ Administer oxygen, if a unit is available and a trained operator is present.
+ Follow basic life support protocols until the ambulance arrives.

hyperventilation

Otherwise known as over-breathing, hyperventilation is usually caused by over-excitement, anxiety, hysteria or strong emotion. In rare cases, hyperventilation may be in response to specific medical conditions (metabolic acidosis, hypercapnoea). In these cases attempts to control the hyperventilation would be counterproductive.

signs

+ Normal or pink skin
+ Rapid deep breathing
+ Gasping respiration or air hunger
+ In severe episodes, patients may experience spasms or cramps in their hands and feet

symptoms

+ A feeling of needing to breathe quickly
+ Anxiety or emotional distress: some people may be having a panic attack and feel like they are having a heart attack and going to die
+ Pins and needles in hands, face and feet

treatment

+ Give reassurance and calm the patient.
+ Encourage the patient to take slow, deep breaths. It may be useful to have the person breathe through one nostril only (closing the mouth), or breathe through pursed lips. This will reduce oxygen intake and allow carbon dioxide levels to normalise.
+ Continue breath coaching the patient until symptoms return to normal.
+ If initial treatment is unsuccessful, seek urgent medical assistance.

asthma

Asthma is a reversible, inflammatory disease of the small airways. When an asthma attack occurs, the muscles in the small airways constrict (bronchospasm), the lining of the airways becomes swollen and inflamed, and excess mucus is produced. Asthma attacks occur in response to certain 'triggers' — so called because they trigger the characteristic inflammatory response in asthma. Asthma triggers include, but are not limited to:

+ pollen
+ fumes
+ smoke (cigarette and wood)
+ dust or dust mite
+ chest infections
+ animal hair/saliva
+ mould
+ distress and anxiety
+ exercise
+ cold air.

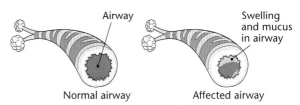

A normal airway compared with a swollen and mucus-filled airway, characteristic of asthma

signs

+ Shortness of breath
+ Increased respiratory rate
+ Shallow respirations
+ Wheezing and coughing
+ Rapid pulse
+ Pale, sweaty skin sometimes becoming blue around the lips, fingertips and earlobes
+ Use of accessory breathing muscles (neck, intercostal and abdominal muscles)
+ Altered state of consciousness

symptoms

+ Anxious and panicky feelings
+ Difficulty speaking — only single words or short phrases possible, or none at all in severe episodes
+ Tiredness, exhaustion

In severe asthma attacks, the audible wheezing may subside as the condition worsens with very little air moving in and out of the lungs. This is an emergency situation. Never assume that a decrease in audible wheeze is a sign of improvement unless breathing also improves.

treatment

+ Sit the patient comfortably upright. Reassure them and remain calm.
+ Give 4 puffs of a blue 'reliever' inhaler (puffer) — use the patient's own, if possible, or use the first aid kit inhaler or borrow one from someone else. Relievers are best given through a spacer, though if a spacer is not available just use the inhaler by itself. Shake the reliever medication and deliver 1 puff into the spacer and have the patient take 4 breaths. Deliver 4 puffs in this fashion.
+ If no spacer is available, shake the inhaler and deliver 1 puff as the patient inhales slowly. Ask them to hold their breath for 4 seconds before taking 4 normal breaths. Repeat the process delivering 4 puffs in total.
+ Wait 4 minutes. If there is little or no improvement, give another 4 puffs.
+ If there is still no improvement, *call an ambulance immediately* and state that the person is having an asthma attack. Continue giving four puffs of reliever medication every 4 minutes until the ambulance arrives.
    — Children: 4 puffs each time is a safe dose.
    — Adults: Up to 6–8 puffs every 5 minutes may be given for a severe attack while waiting for the ambulance.
+ If the patient loses consciousness at any stage, place them on their side, make sure their airway is clear and monitor their breathing and circulation. Should it be necessary, start CPR.

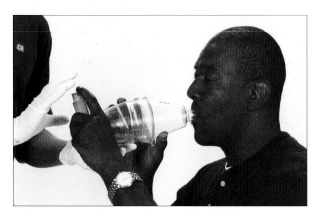

Administering reliever medication through a spacer

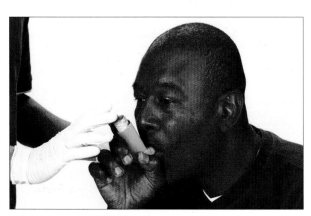

Administering reliever medication without a spacer

what if this is the first attack of asthma?

+ If this is the first episode of breathing difficulty (i.e. the patient has not been diagnosed with asthma) and the patient collapses, call an ambulance immediately.
+ Administer reliever medication as described above, while waiting for medical help to arrive.
+ It is extremely unlikely that reliever medication will adversely affect someone who turns out not to have asthma.

suffocation

Suffocation is oxygen deprivation that may lead to death.

treatment

+ Call an ambulance.
+ Follow DRABCD (see Chapter 3).
+ Remove the patient from danger without placing yourself at risk.
+ Open and clear the airway of the unconscious patient.
+ Start EAR (see Chapter 4) delivering 5 breaths before checking for the carotid pulse.
+ If there is no pulse, start CPR (see Chapter 5) and continue until the patient recovers or medical help arrives.

smoke/ gas inhalation

Gas or smoke inhalation can cause a respiratory emergency. Circumstances as simple as standing next to a car exhaust can reduce the amount of oxygen getting to the lungs. Other circumstances where people may inhale dangerous gases or smoke are house fires, painting, working in confined spaces or risk-taking behaviour. The patient may experience altered consciousness or may even die.

treatment

+ Follow DRABCD (see Chapter 3).
+ Ensure the area is safe (and adequately ventilated) before entering.
+ Remove the patient from the dangerous area to a safe place with plenty of fresh air.
+ Calm the patient and reassure them.
+ Administer oxygen, if an oxygen unit and qualified personnel are available.
+ Start EAR and CPR as necessary, taking care to use a barrier device for EAR to avoid poisoning by absorption (see Chapter 14).

respiratory emergencies

chapter eight

NOTE:
If the patient is unconscious and not breathing, ensure you use a barrier device when performing EAR to avoid possible poisoning by absorption.

allergic reactions

Allergic reactions can occur following exposure to certain allergens, such as drugs, dust, animal dander (feathers, hair etc), pollens, insect stings and some foods (e.g. peanuts, shellfish). Severe allergies can be life-threatening if a patient goes into anaphylactic shock (see Chapter 7).

NOTE:
Patients with severe allergies may be wearing a MedicAlert tag (necklace or bracelet).

signs

+ Reddened skin or a rash, which may be on just one part of the body or all over it
+ Raised itchy lumps or hives (urticaria) on the skin
+ Swelling of the tongue and constriction of the throat
+ Swelling of the face
+ Wheezing
+ Vomiting
+ Unconsciousness

symptoms

+ Difficulty breathing
+ Fear and anxiety
+ Nausea
+ Feeling dizzy or faint

treatment

+ Rest and reassure the patient.
+ Help the patient into a comfortable position. If the patient wants to lie down, elevate their legs.
+ If the allergy is caused by an insect (e.g. bee), treat as for that insect bite (see Chapter 15).
+ If the reaction is severe or over the entire body, call an ambulance and treat for shock.
+ If the reaction is localised, seek medical advice.
+ Patients in anaphylaxis require adrenaline, and those with severe allergies or a history of anaphylaxis usually carry adrenaline in a self-injecting pen (an EpiPen). Assist the patient self-inject adrenaline, if possible.
+ If the patient becomes unconscious at any stage, make sure their airway is clear and monitor their breathing and circulation. Should it be necessary, start CPR.

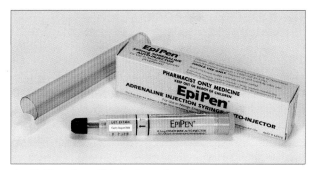

An EpiPen for self-injecting adrenaline

chest injuries

Any disruption to the integrity of the chest wall is a serious condition because of the likelihood of damage to the lungs, which will compromise breathing, as well as the heart and major vessels. Chest injuries, such as penetrating chest wounds or traumatic pneumothorax will lead to respiratory distress and require intervention by the rescuer.

spontaneous pneumothorax

Two membranes line the outside of the lungs, one of which adheres to the inside of the chest wall with relative negative pressure in between. Therefore, the lungs follow the movement of the rib cage and take air in and expel it as the chest wall expands and contracts, respectively. Pneumothorax is the build-up of air in the space between these two layers/membranes. This may occur spontaneously, from blunt or penetrating trauma (see Chapter 11), secondary to an underlying lung disease or from excessive pressure build-up around the lungs (tension pneumothorax). Usually, this will lead to a degree of respiratory distress, depending on the size of the pneumothorax. Sometimes pneumothorax can reduce the space available in the chest cavity for the heart and lungs. Eventually, this can put pressure on the lungs and heart, leading to compromised respiratory and cardiac function and may result in death.

signs

+ Respiratory distress
+ Shallow rapid respirations
+ Increased heart rate

symptoms

+ Pain and tenderness at the site of the injury
+ Pain while breathing or coughing

treatment

+ Call an ambulance.
+ Rest and reassure the patient.
+ Position the patient as upright as possible, leaning slightly towards the injured side.
+ Administer oxygen if an oxygen unit and qualified personnel are available.

flail segment/chest

When a rib is broken in more than one place, it often appears to be floating as it is held in place only by the intercostal muscles and tissues of the chest wall. Due to the different pressures within the lungs, the floating segment of rib will move in the opposite direction to the rest of the ribs — known as paradoxical respirations. Hence, when the patient breathes in and their chest moves out, the flail or floating segment moves inwards. This causes severe pain and reduces the amount of lung space available for air to move into. A flail chest is often associated with pneumothorax, lung contusion (bruising) and hypoxia and these complications make it a potentially life-threatening condition.

signs

+ Respiratory distress
+ Shallow rapid respirations
+ Increased heart rate
+ Bruising or swelling of the chest wall

symptoms

+ Pain and tenderness at the site of the injury
+ Pain while breathing or coughing

treatment

+ Call an ambulance.
+ Follow DRABCD.
+ Rest and reassure the patient.
+ Position the patient as upright as possible, leaning slightly towards the injured side.
+ Give the patient oxygen if an oxygen unit and trained personnel are available.
+ To reduce the movement of the flail segment, pad the wound and secure around the chest wall with a broad triangular bandage. If these are unavailable, place a pillow over the site of the injury and ask the patient to hold it firmly onto their chest.

winding

Patients who have been winded may require first aid, though this is rarely a respiratory emergency. Winding is the experience of having the breath knocked out of you and typically occurs after a blow to the stomach or back around the solar plexus (a cluster of sympathetic nerves behind the stomach influencing respiration).

signs

+ Difficulty breathing
+ Inability to speak
+ Vomiting

symptoms

+ Nausea

treatment

+ Reassure the patient.
+ Help the patient into a comfortable position.
+ Remain with the person until the breathing difficulty resolves.
+ If the breathing difficulty does not improve in a few minutes, seek medical attention.
+ Lay the unconscious patient on their side in the lateral position, ensuring the airway remains clear and monitor the patient's breathing.

revision

1. Which of the following is *not* true?
   a) The normal breathing rate for adults is 12–16 breaths per minute.
   b) The normal breathing rate for children is 30 breaths per minute.
   c) Abnormal breathing rates for adults are <10 breaths per minute and >20 breaths per minute.
   d) Abnormal breathing rates for children are <15 breaths per minute and >25 breaths per minute.

2. Complete the following sentence about drowning.

   Drowning is death by ……………… from immersion in ……………… or other ………………

3. What are the signs of laryngeal spasm?

   a) _____

   b) _____

   c) _____

   d) _____

4. How would you treat a person with hyperventilation?

   _____

   _____

   _____

5. How is asthma defined?

   _____

   _____

6. Which of the following statements relating to asthma is *not* true?
   a) Never assume that a decrease in audible wheeze is a sign of improvement in asthma unless breathing also improves.
   b) Asthma attacks occur in response to certain 'triggers'.
   c) Reliever medications are best delivered through a spacer.
   d) If a spacer is not available for use with reliever medication, improvise by constructing a make-shift spacer.

7. Complete the following sentence regarding what happens during a pneumothorax.

   Pneumothorax is the build-up of ……………… in the space between the two membrane layers around the

   ………………

8. What are the signs of a spontaneous pneumothorax?

   a) _____

   b) _____

   c) _____

9. What happens during respirations in a flail chest?

   _____

   _____

   _____

Answers appear in Appendix 8.

cardiovascular emergencies

learning outcomes

Perform first aid to manage cardiovascular emergencies.

+ Detail the causes of cardiovascular emergencies.
+ Detail the risk factors associated with cardiovascular disease.
+ Demonstrate how perfusion status is assessed.
+ Detail the signs and symptoms of and treatment for a patient with angina.
+ Detail the signs and symptoms of and treatment for a patient who has suffered a heart attack.
+ Detail the signs and symptoms of and treatment for a patient who has suffered a cerebrovascular accident (stroke).
+ Detail the signs and symptoms of and treatment for a patient with congestive/chronic heart failure.
+ Detail the signs and symptoms of and treatment for a patient with a suspected deep vein thrombosis.
+ Detail the signs and symptoms of and treatment for patients who have cardiovascular emergencies when diving.

how you may be assessed

underpinning knowledge

A number of written or oral questions may be asked relating to assessing perfusion status, the causes of and risk factors associated with cardiovascular disease and the signs and symptoms of and treatment for angina, heart attack, cerebrovascular accidents or strokes, chronic heart failure, deep vein thrombosis and emergencies when diving. Examples have been included at the end of the chapter.

practical demonstration

You may be asked to show how you would assess a patient's perfusion status. You may be asked to show how you would identify and treat a patient suffering from a cardiovascular emergency.

scenario

You may be required to demonstrate how you would identify one or more patients suffering from a cardiovascular emergency.

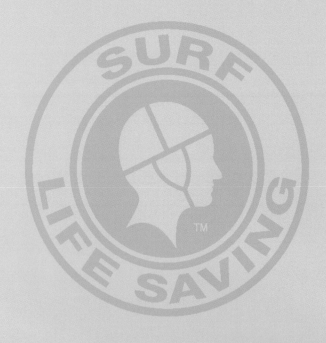

Cardiovascular emergencies encompass diseases affecting the circulatory system. Those most likely to be seen and to require management are cardiac chest pain and cardiac arrest. These may be due to underlying cardiovascular disease or from other causes, though management is the same regardless of the cause. Early notification of the ambulance service will improve patient management and ensure the best possible outcome for the patient.

cardiovascular disease

Cardiovascular disease is the term used for diseases of the circulatory system. Cardiovascular disease is more common in individuals with established risk factors, some of which are modifiable, while others are non-modifiable, as shown in the following table.

From a very early age, fatty deposits become embedded in the walls of arteries forming 'plaque', rather like sediment clogging up an old water pipe. As the plaque develops and becomes thicker, the interior diameter of the vessels (lumen) narrows, decreasing blood flow to the tissues on the far side (distal) of the plaque. This process (atherosclerosis) can occur in arteries throughout the body and is classified according to where it occurs:

RISK FACTORS THAT CAN'T BE CHANGED (NON-MODIFIABLE)

- Family history (heredity)
- Being male
- Increasing age

RISK FACTORS THAT CAN BE CHANGED (MODIFIABLE)

- High cholesterol levels (hypercholesterolaemia)
- High blood sugar (diabetes)
- High blood pressure (hypertension)
- Elevated homocysteine levels
- Smoking
- Excessive alcohol consumption
- Obesity (BMI*>30) and overweight (BMI*>25)
- Psychosocial factors (e.g. depression, anxiety, social isolation)
- Physical inactivity (<3 half-hour sessions of aerobic activity/week)

* BMI = body mass index kg/m^2

+ coronary artery disease (CAD) affects the arteries around the heart, which supply the heart muscle with blood. CAD may cause angina (cramps of the heart muscle due to a disruption in the blood supply) and, in severe cases, myocardial infarction (MI), which may be fatal

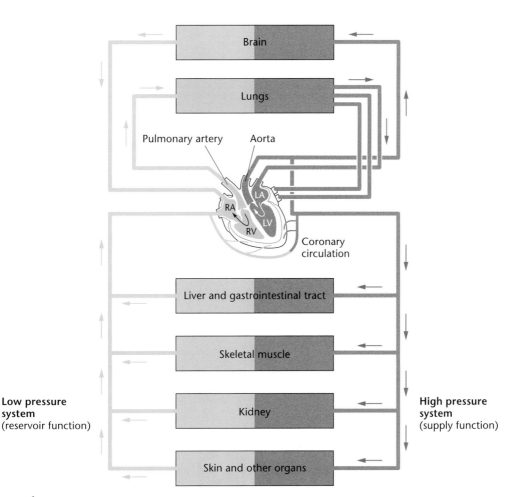

The cardiovascular system

+ cerebrovascular disease affects arteries in the brain. Restriction of the blood supply to the brain is known as stroke. Stroke may be caused by the complete blockage (occlusion) of a blood vessel (ischaemic cerebrovascular disease) or by bleeding into the brain (haemorrhage)
+ peripheral vascular disease affects arteries in the limb (usually the legs, causing leg cramps when walking).

Plaques can rupture leading to bleeding and thrombosis (a blood clot forms in the vessel). The clot may occlude the vessel (thrombosis), and fragments of the clot may break off and occlude arteries elsewhere in the body (thromboembolism). This is a medical emergency when it occurs in the heart, lungs or brain.

Chronic heart failure is the inability of the heart to pump blood efficiently, leading to a back-up of blood and fluid throughout the body.

assessing perfusion status

The perfusion status assessment is made up of four observations which, when taken in the context of the patient's presenting problem, help determine whether the cardiovascular system is functioning adequately. Any patient who has changes to two or more of the following categories (pulse, consciousness, skin colour, skin temperature) should be considered to be less than adequately perfused. Such a person is regarded to be 'actual time-critical' (see Chapter 22) and in urgent need of medical attention for survival.

pulse

Using the pads of two or three fingers (but not the thumb), feel for either the carotid or radial artery. Count the pulse for 15 seconds and multiply by 4 to give the patient's pulse rate per minute. The normal pulse rate for an adult is 60–100 beats per minute. A faster or slower rate than this may indicate the heart is not pumping as efficiently as normal, or that there is not enough oxygen being supplied to the tissues.

state of consciousness

See Chapter 10 on conditions affecting level of consciousness and Appendix 5 for a detailed description of how to assess a patient's level of consciousness.

Under normal circumstances, a patient should be alert and orientated in time and place. An altered level of consciousness may indicate a lack of oxygen delivered to the brain, which may occur if the heart is not pumping effectively.

skin colour and temperature

Observe the patient's skin colour and feel it for warmth. An adult's skin is normally warm (depending on environmental factors), pink and dry. If the patient's skin is pale or cyanosed (blue looking), or cool and clammy (excluding environmental factors), it may indicate that the body is compensating for something and supplying only the vital organs with oxygen. Pale, cool, clammy skin is indicative of reduced blood supply to the skin.

angina

Angina refers to the chest pain and associated symptoms felt when there is a decrease in the blood flow and oxygen delivery to the heart muscle. This usually occurs in response to known stressors, such as exercise and stress.

It can be very difficult to distinguish angina from chest pain originating from other sources (e.g. severe indigestion). If in doubt, always treat as if the pain is a cardiac emergency until proven otherwise. Any chest pain lasting over 10 minutes must be treated as a cardiac emergency.

NOTE:
• Check the patient for a MedicAlert tag.
• Chest pain (angina) lasting >10 minutes must be treated as a cardiac emergency.

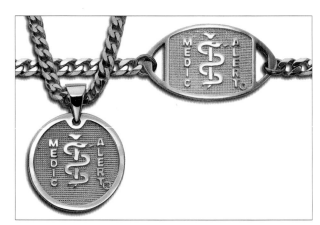

MedicAlert tag on necklace and bracelet

signs
+ Shortness of breath
+ Vomiting
+ Paleness and profuse sweating
+ Person may be wearing a nitrate skin patch (usually on hair-free skin on upper arm or chest)

symptoms
+ Pain, tightness or heaviness in the centre of the chest, which may radiate down either arm, although commonly the left, and into the neck, back or jaw
+ Nausea
+ Anxiety and emotional distress

NOTE:
Patients may experience any or all of the above symptoms.

treatment

✚ Rest and reassure the patient — ensure that they stop all physical activity.

✚ Place the patient in the most comfortable position — usually semi-reclining.

✚ If you consider the circumstances require it, advise and assist the patient loosen tight clothing around their neck and chest.

✚ Administer oxygen via a facemask, if an oxygen unit and trained personnel are available.

✚ Ask the patient about any medical conditions. If they suffer from angina, encourage them to take their own medication, if available (nitrate sprays, tablets placed under the tongue).

✚ If this is the first presentation or pain does not resolve with the patient's own medication and/or rest, call for an ambulance.

✚ Patients experiencing chest pain may deteriorate rapidly. Monitor the patient closely. Be prepared to administer CPR (see Chapter 5).

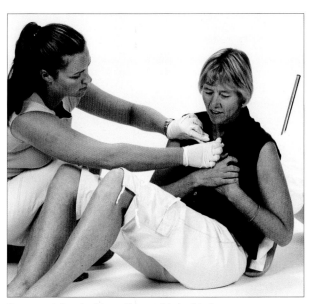

Loosen tight clothing, if you think this is necessary

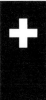

NOTE:
Patients who suffer from angina usually carry their own medication and do not need to see a doctor if the pain resolves within 10 minutes after rest and/or medication.

heart attack

When one of the arteries supplying the heart (coronary arteries) becomes blocked, there is no blood flow to the tissues beyond the blockage. Oxygen deprivation results in death or permanent damage to heart muscle cells (myocardial tissue) causing a heart attack.

Cardiac arrest is defined as the absence of breathing and a pulse. This can have several causes, including cardiac disease, respiratory failure, trauma and drug overdose or poisoning. Irrespective of the cause, the principles of management are the same.

The vital organs of the body require a constant supply of oxygen. Without oxygen, the brain cells will begin to die within 3–5 minutes; the heart will stop pumping effectively within 5–10 minutes. No matter what the cause of cardiac arrest, the result is that blood flow and oxygen delivery throughout the body stops.

signs and symptoms

✚ The same as those of angina, although often more severe, and the pain does not usually resolve with rest or the patient's own medication

✚ Unconsciousness

✚ Absence of a palpable carotid pulse

✚ Shortness of breath or absent respiration

✚ Cold, pale or blue (cyanosed) skin

treatment

✚ Send someone to call an ambulance.

✚ Rest and reassure the conscious patient — ensure they stop all physical activity.

✚ Place the patient in the most comfortable position — usually semi-reclining.

✚ If you consider the circumstances require it, advise and assist the patient loosen tight clothing around their neck and chest.

✚ Ask the patient about any medical conditions. If they suffer from angina, encourage them to take their own medication, if available.

✚ If the patient collapses suddenly, place them in the lateral position, make sure their airway is clear and monitor breathing and circulation. Should it be necessary, start CPR.

✚ For the unconscious patient, remember the 'chain of survival', early access, early CPR, early defibrillation and early advanced life support (see Chapter 4).

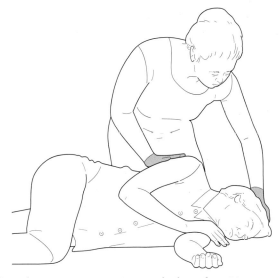

Place the unconscious patient in the lateral position

cerebrovascular accident (stroke)

A cerebrovascular accident (CVA) is also called a *stroke*. Stroke is the most common disease of the nervous system and ranks as the third leading cause of death throughout the world. It can affect people in all age groups, but is more prevalent in people between 75 and 85 years of age. Very minor strokes followed by full functional recovery are called transient ischaemic attacks (TIAs).

Stroke is caused by an interruption of the blood supply to parts of the brain (from vessel occlusion or haemorrhage), restricting blood flow to areas of the brain with subsequent cell death (infarction). The brain is extremely sensitive to alterations in oxygen supply and permanent damage and cell death can occur within 3–5 minutes of restricted blood flow.

signs and symptoms

The type of damage will depend on the area of the brain that has been affected, and this depends on which cerebral vessels are involved. The following are the general signs and symptoms associated with a stroke, but, depending on the extent of the damage to the brain, there may be only a few or multiple presenting signs.

motor abnormalities

+ Loss of muscle strength, usually on one side of the body (hemiplegia)
+ Loss of co-ordination
+ Facial paralysis, drooping eyelids, drooling
+ Inability or difficulty swallowing

sensory abnormalities

+ Loss of sensation (numbness)
+ Altered sensation (tingling)
+ Loss of balance

speech abnormalities

+ Loss of speech
+ Slurred speech
+ Dysphasia (problems using or understanding language)

respiration

+ May be unimpaired
+ Potential for airway compromise
+ Potential for impaired respiration if the respiratory centre in the brainstem is affected

conscious state

+ May be unimpaired, despite obvious and severe symptoms
+ Confusion
+ Seizures
+ Altered mood or personality change
+ Altered consciousness — sleepy, lethargic or comatose

general abnormalities

+ Headaches
+ Incontinence
+ Nausea and vomiting
+ Elevated blood pressure

A simple tool to identify whether a patient has had a stroke is the Cincinnati pre-hospital stroke scale. When used by physicians, this scale can help select patients suitable for therapy designed to break down blood clots (thrombolytic therapy), which must start within 3 hours of the vascular event. Time is critical for stroke patients and they require urgent transport to hospital.

CINCINNATI PRE-HOSPITAL STROKE SCALE

Facial droop (have patient show teeth or smile)
Normal: both sides move equally well
Abnormal: one side of face does not move as well as the other side

---

Arm drift (patient closes eyes and holds both arms out for 10 seconds)
Normal: both arms move the same or both arms do not move at all
Abnormal: one arm does not move or one arm drifts down compared with the other

---

Speech (have the patient say "you can't teach an old dog new tricks")
Normal: patient uses the correct words with no slurring
Abnormal: patient slurs words, uses inappropriate words, or is unable to speak

---

treatment

+ Have someone call an ambulance immediately. A suspected stroke should be treated as seriously as a suspected heart attack.
+ Administer oxygen via a facemask, if an oxygen unit and qualified personnel are available.
+ Constantly reassure the alert patient, even if they cannot communicate.
+ Care for any paralysed limbs — place the patient in a comfortable position (when moving the patient, be careful not to cause injury to paralysed limbs).
+ Place an unconscious patient in the lateral position. Make sure their airway is clear and monitor the patient's breathing and circulation. Should it be necessary, start CPR (see Chapter 5).
+ Be prepared for respiratory failure — even when conscious, stroke patients can have a diminished airway due to loss of the cough and swallow reflexes.

congestive or chronic heart failure

When the heart is unable to pump sufficient blood throughout the body, circulatory congestion occurs with a back-up of blood volume and swelling in some areas of the body (oedema). This can develop as a result of damage to the heart (heart attack), as well as numerous other causes.

Congestive heart failure is almost invariably a chronic, long-term problem. The term 'heart failure' refers to the ability to pump blood effectively, rather than the heart stopping, as in a heart attack.

signs

+ Acute shortness of breath
+ Noisy gurgling breathing
+ Rapid or irregular pulse
+ Cough
+ Grey, blue (cyanosed) or pale and clammy skin
+ Swelling of the legs and/or ankles (oedema)
+ Decreased urine output

symptoms

+ Fatigue, faintness
+ Nausea and vomiting

treatment

+ Call an ambulance immediately.
+ Rest and reassure the patient.
+ Sit the patient upright (do not elevate the legs).
+ Loosen any tight clothing.
+ If the patient becomes unconscious at any stage, place them on their side, make sure their airway is clear and monitor their breathing and circulation. Should it be necessary, start CPR (see Chapter 5).

deep vein thrombosis

Deep vein thrombosis (DVT) is a condition characterised by blood clots in deep veins, typically involving the legs. Clots interfere with circulation and carry a risk of embolism, whereby small pieces of the clot break off and lodge in small arteries throughout the body. This typically involves the heart, lungs or brain, causing tissue damage and, potentially, death.

DVT is associated with established risk factors, such as prolonged periods of immobility (e.g. long trips, prolonged bed rest), recent trauma, major fractures or surgery, taking oestrogen therapy (including the oral contraceptive pill) and recent childbirth.

signs and symptoms

+ Pain and tenderness in one limb
+ Red limb that is warm to the touch
+ Sudden-onset swelling (oedema) of the limb

treatment

+ Observe the patient for signs of respiratory difficulty, suggestive of pulmonary embolism. Monitor breathing and circulation in these patients and perform EAR and CPR as necessary, after calling for an ambulance.
+ All patients with symptoms suggestive of DVT should be sent to a hospital emergency department for assessment.

cardiovascular diving emergencies

There are two main types of diving emergencies:

+ *air embolism*: the more common condition that a first aider will need to treat — caused by a too rapid and uncontrolled ascent, usually causing unconsciousness with a high probability of drowning
+ *decompression illness*: usually presenting after the dive and less likely for the first aider to need to treat. Symptoms usually develop up to 48 hours after the dive, especially if air travel is involved within this time frame.

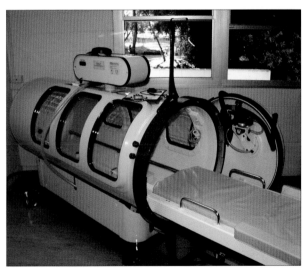

Hyperbaric chamber: commonly used in dive emergencies

signs and symptoms

air embolism

+ Dizziness and disorientation
+ Altered level of consciousness
+ Weakness or paralysis
+ Chest pain
+ Bloody froth from the mouth or nose
+ Blurred or disturbed vision
+ Shock

decompression illness

+ Fatigue
+ Itchy skin
+ Joint pain
+ Coughing

- Abdominal pain
- Disorientation
- Numbness or tingling
- Paralysis or muscle weakness
- Shortness of breath
- Shock

treatment

- Immediately place the patient flat on their back, with the head level with the heart. Do not elevate the head.
- Follow DRABCD (see Chapter 3).

- Resuscitate the patient, if necessary (see Chapters 4, 5).
- Administer oxygen in the highest concentration possible:
  — anaesthetic mask with airbag and oxygen reservoir bag, if necessary
  — deliver oxygen direct to the diver's demand valve, if a connection is available.
- Reassure the patient.
- Remain with the patient and send others for help.

revision

1. List the non-modifiable risk factors for cardiovascular disease:

   a) _____ b) _____ c) _____

2. What is atherosclerosis called when it occurs:

   a) in the vessels around the heart? _____

   b) in the vessels in the brain? _____

   c) in the vessels in the limbs? _____

3. Which four observations should you take to assess perfusion status?

   a) _____ b) _____

   c) _____ d) _____

4. Complete the following sentence about angina.

   Pain, ... or heaviness in the centre of the ...., which may radiate down either ...., although commonly the left, and into the ...., back or jaw.

5. What is the definition of cardiac arrest?

   _____

   _____

6. Which of the following statements about stroke is *not* true?
   a) It is the second leading cause of death worldwide.
   b) Very minor strokes followed by full functional recovery are called transient ischaemic attacks.
   c) The damage resulting from a stroke depends on the area of the brain affected.
   d) Stroke may result from vessel occlusion or haemorrhage.

7. Which three criteria are assessed in the Cincinnati pre-hospital stroke scale?

   a) _____ b) _____ c) _____

8. List 5 signs of congestive heart failure:

   a) _____ b) _____ c) _____

   d) _____ e) _____

9. List the signs and symptoms of deep vein thrombosis:

   a) _____

   b) _____

   c) _____

10. List the two most common cardiovascular diving emergencies, and indicate which is more likely to be seen by the first aider.

    a) _____

    b) _____

Answers appear in Appendix 8.

conditions affecting level of consciousness

learning outcomes

Perform first aid to manage conditions with affected levels of consciousness.

- Describe how to assess level of consciousness.
- Demonstrate appropriate care for the unconscious patient.
- Demonstrate appropriate treatment for a patient who has a convulsive epileptic seizure.
- Demonstrate appropriate treatment for a patient who suffers a febrile convulsion.
- Detail the types of diabetes.
- Detail the signs and symptoms of and treatment for a patient suffering from hypoglycaemia.
- Detail the signs and symptoms of and treatment for a patient suffering from hyperglycaemia.
- Detail the signs and symptoms of and treatment for a patient who has fainted.
- Detail the signs and symptoms of and treatment for a patient with an altered state of consciousness after sustaining a head injury.

how you may be assessed

underpinning knowledge

A number of written or oral questions may be asked relating to levels of consciousness, unconsciousness, epileptic seizures, febrile convulsions, diabetes, hypoglycaemia, hyperglycaemia, fainting and head injuries. Examples have been included at the end of the chapter.

practical demonstration

You be asked to demonstrate how you would assess a patient's level of consciousness. You may be asked to show how you would treat an unconscious patient. You may be asked to demonstrate how you would treat a patient during and after an epileptic seizure. You may be asked to demonstrate how you would treat a patient suffering from febrile convulsions. You may be asked to demonstrate how you would recognise and treat a patient suffering from hypoglycaemia or hyperglycaemia. You may be asked to demonstrate how you would treat a patient who has fainted. You may be asked to show how you would treat a patient who has sustained a head injury.

scenario

You may be required to demonstrate how you would identify one or more patients suffering from an altered level of consciousness.

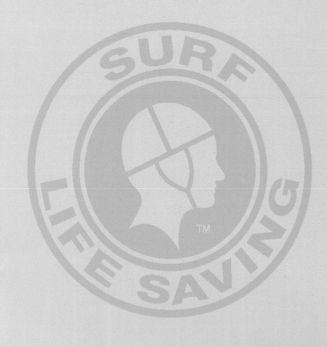

Consciousness reflects a person's responsiveness to stimuli. Consciousness ranges from full awareness/responsiveness and orientation in time and place to unconsciousness, being unaware of one's surroundings and unresponsive to stimulation. It is important to determine a patient's level of consciousness, as this will determine your care of the patient.

assessment of level of consciousness

A thorough clinical assessment involves an accurate, standardised and repeatable measure of consciousness. This is best achieved through the Glasgow Coma Scale (GCS; see Appendix 5).

care of the unconscious patient

The main role of the first aider is to protect the unconscious patient's airway from obstruction and prevent further injury.

causes of altered consciousness/ unconsciousness

The causes of alterations in the state of consciousness can be recalled by the acronym 'AEIOU TIPS'. This stands for:

+ **A** alcohol
+ **E** epilepsy
+ **I** insulin overdose or underdose (diabetes)
+ **O** overdose (drugs, poisons)
+ **U** uraemia (renal failure)
+ **T** trauma, toxic fumes
+ **I** infection
+ **P** psychiatric conditions (e.g. catatonic states)
+ **S** stroke, shock.

treatment of altered consciousness/ unconsciousness

Treatment of patients with altered consciousness or the unconscious patient will depend on the primary cause, as outlined in this chapter. However, the core treatment principles are listed below.

+ Follow DRABCD (see Chapter 3).
+ Send someone to call an ambulance.

+ Manage any injuries appropriately.
+ Assess the scene for likely causes of altered consciousness/unconsciousness, but do not leave the patient.

NOTE:
An unconscious patient should be assumed to have a spinal injury until proven otherwise. Therefore, be very careful when rolling and moving the patient

epilepsy

Many conditions may cause individuals to have isolated seizures (e.g. head injury, after poisoning, cardiac arrest, etc), though only recurrent seizures are diagnosed as epilepsy. The characteristic seizures, or fits, in epilepsy are due to the disruption in normal brain functioning with abnormal discharge of activity causing disturbances in consciousness and/or movement. Seizures are described as being generalised when they affect the entire brain or partial when they only affect one side of, or a focal point in, the brain.

convulsive seizures

Convulsive or generalised tonic clonic seizures are characterised by loss of consciousness with stiffening of the body (tonic phase) and jerking of the limbs (clonic phase). Seizures usually last from one to three minutes. Following these seizures (previously called grand mal seizures), the person may be very tired and wish to rest or sleep, have a headache and be confused or disoriented. They should be referred for further medical assessment.

treatment

+ Remain calm and stay with the patient.
+ Do not move the patient with known epilepsy unless they are in danger, e.g. from a roadway, or near fire or water. Patients should remain seated if seizures occur in prams/strollers, wheelchairs or car seats. Other patients should be placed in the recovery position on their side.

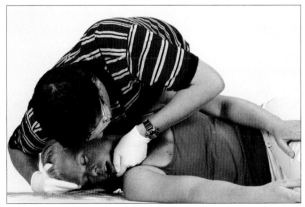

If necessary, check the person's airway and breathing on recovery from a seizure. Call an ambulance if the person has difficulty breathing

- Remove nearby objects to prevent injury to the patient.
- Place something soft under the patient's head.
- Time the seizure.
- Loosen any tight clothing the patient is wearing.
- Do not restrain the person.
- Do not put anything in the person's mouth.
- If the patient vomits, place them in the lateral position immediately. Otherwise, do so on recovery.
- Cover with a blanket or a sheet in case there is incontinence, due to loss of bladder or bowel control.
- Reassure the person until they have recovered fully.

NOTE:
Call an ambulance if:
- a seizure lasts longer than 5 minutes, or is longer than usual for an individual
- it is a person's first seizure
- one seizure is followed quickly by another
- the person is injured
- the person has breathing difficulties after the seizure
- the person is pregnant
- the person has diabetes.

non-convulsive seizures

Partial seizures affect a specific area of the brain and, as such, the type of seizure depends on the area involved (e.g. one limb may stiffen or jerk, the person may experience an alteration in taste or smell or the person may engage in stereotypic behaviour such as picking at hair or clothes, walking, grunting or lip smacking, etc). There may be some alteration of consciousness and the person may appear unresponsive or confused. Absence seizures (previously called petit mal seizures) are typically seen in children, and are characterised by a loss of consciousness that appears like daydreaming or poor concentration.

treatment

- Remain calm and stay with the patient. This is the only treatment necessary for absence seizures.
- Time the seizure.
- Do not restrain the person.
- Reassure the person until they have recovered fully.
- Call an ambulance if a partial seizure lasts longer than 15 minutes.

febrile convulsions

These are convulsions occurring in children under the age of 5 years, in association with any illness that produces a rapid rise in body temperature. Children have a lower seizure threshold and are, consequently, more sensitive to changes in brain activity than adults. Febrile convulsions do not mean the child has or will develop epilepsy, which are recurrent seizures not associated with high temperatures.

treatment

- Remain calm — the sight of a child convulsing can be very distressing.
- Reassure the parents or carers. Although frightening, febrile convulsions in children resolve quickly and are not life-threatening.
- Remove the child from any danger. Do not restrain the child or attempt to force the mouth open, as this may cause further damage.
- Remove any excessive clothing, but do not let the child become chilled.
- Seek medical advice and follow their directions during and after recovery, assess breathing and perform EAR, if necessary (see Chapter 4).

NOTE:
Call an ambulance if:
- the seizures do not stop when the child's temperature has been lowered
- resuscitation is necessary.

diabetes

Diabetes is a condition characterised by the body's inability to maintain blood sugar levels due to lack of insulin (which decreases elevated blood sugar levels) or tissue resistance to insulin.

There are three main types of diabetes:

- *Type 1 diabetes:* an autoimmune condition where the insulin-secreting cells in the pancreas are destroyed. This condition typically presents before the age of 30 years, though usually early in childhood. Previously known as insulin-dependent diabetes, patients with Type 1 diabetes require insulin-replacement injections to survive.
- *Type 2 diabetes:* generally affects people over the age of 40 years and accounts for around 85% of all cases of diabetes. Lifestyle factors (lack of exercise and obesity) are the biggest contributing factors in developing Type 2 diabetes. In Type 2 diabetes, rising insulin resistance results in the insulin-secreting cells in the pancreas becoming exhausted, resulting in lower insulin levels. Previously known as non-insulin-dependent diabetes, this condition may be controlled with diet and exercise, oral medication, or may require insulin-replacement therapy.
- *Gestational diabetes:* occurs during pregnancy and does not usually persist long after delivery. Most cases can be controlled by a good diet and exercise, though some women will require insulin.

People with diabetes are at risk of episodes of loss of consciousness due to:

- excessive lowering of blood sugar level, or hypoglycaemia. This occurs very quickly and needs urgent medical attention, as brain damage and death may occur within hours

✚ very high blood sugar levels, or hyperglycaemia. This usually occurs more slowly, and is less likely to be seen by a first aider.

In any case of sudden, unexpected and unexplained loss of consciousness, there is a possibility that the person may have diabetes. Look for signs of injection marks on the lower abdomen or the front of the thighs. Always look for a MedicAlert tag — this may be on the wrist or ankle or around the neck — or a diabetes ID card.

signs of hypoglycaemia

✚ Pallor
✚ Excessive sweating
✚ Rapid pulse
✚ Seizures
✚ Altered state of consciousness or loss of consciousness
✚ The patient may be wearing a MedicAlert tag

symptoms of hypoglycaemia

✚ Feeling shaky or tremulous
✚ Anxiety
✚ Dizziness and loss of concentration
✚ Confusion, such that the patient is not able to help/treat themselves

treatment for hypoglycaemia

If the patient is unconscious:

✚ Call an ambulance immediately.
✚ Follow DRABCD.
✚ Give the patient oxygen if an oxygen unit and trained personnel are available .
✚ Do not try to give the patient sugary substances by mouth.

If the patient is conscious:

✚ Help the patient take some foods with fast-acting sugar, such as a sachet or lumps of sugar, juice, glucose gel or soft drinks. Jellybeans and other sweets should be given as a last resort as they take time to dissolve. People with diabetes will usually carry suitable snacks with them.
✚ On recovery, make sure the patient eats a sandwich (or similar high-carbohydrate food) and drinks some juice.

signs of hyperglycaemia

✚ Hot, dry skin
✚ Breath smells like acetone (sweet apples or nail-polish remover)
✚ Frequent urination
✚ Loss of consciousness
✚ The patient may be wearing a MedicAlert tag

symptoms of hyperglycaemia

✚ Thirst
✚ Hunger
✚ Blurred vision
✚ Tiredness

treatment for hyperglycaemia

✚ Call an ambulance immediately, as hyperglycaemia is harder to diagnose than hypoglycaemia and insulin injections are required.
✚ Follow DRABCD (see Chapter 3).
✚ Give the patient oxygen if an oxygen unit and trained personnel are available.
✚ Do not give the patient sugary foods.
✚ Place the unconscious patient in the lateral position and monitor the airway, breathing and circulation.

fainting (syncope)

Fainting, or syncope, is the term used to describe a condition of sudden, brief, loss of consciousness, followed by a rapid and full recovery. Fainting should not be confused with loss of consciousness from shock or any other cause.

Some conditions that may cause fainting include:

✚ standing for prolonged periods in hot weather or in a hot shower
✚ the sight of needles, particularly prior to or after an injection
✚ the sight of blood
✚ extreme hunger or low blood sugar
✚ pain.

Frequently, there are associated signs and symptoms (warning signs) preceding the loss of consciousness.

signs

✚ Sweating
✚ Pale appearance
✚ Collapse

symptoms

✚ Light-headedness and dizziness
✚ Nausea
✚ Feeling of anxiety

treatment

✚ If the patient is unconscious, put them in the lateral position and monitor airway, breathing and circulation.
✚ If conscious, lay the patient flat without a pillow, keep the patient's head level with the heart and raise their legs. If the patient does not lie down, there may be loss of consciousness, depression of breathing and perhaps a brief convulsion. A fall may cause injury.

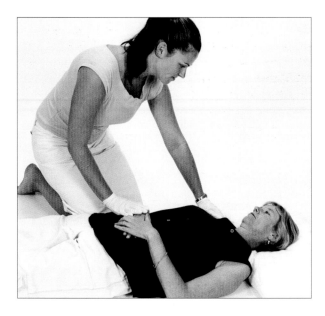

When the patient is placed horizontally, recovery is usually rapid — consciousness is regained, colour returns to the face, normal breathing resumes and the pulse rate returns to normal. If recovery does not occur, send for medical help, as there may be another cause for the loss of consciousness.

head injury

Head injury is common in patients following trauma due to contact and/or acceleration/deceleration forces. The most frequent cause of head injuries are motor vehicle accidents, but the first aider should be aware of other causes, such as falls (being dumped from a wave into shallow water) and assaults.

The brain is surrounded by cerebrospinal fluid and contained within the skull to protect it against such forces. However, the inflexible, bony skull can exacerbate brain injuries if there is swelling, because the pressure within the skull increases, further compressing the already traumatised brain.

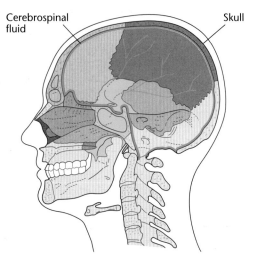

The brain is protected by cerebrospinal fluid and the bony skull

primary brain injury

+ *Concussion:* this is a transient alteration in cerebral function. It is usually associated with loss of or reduced consciousness. This is a result of the brain being shaken excessively or violently, usually by a blow to the head.
+ *Contusion:* this involves various degrees of bruising of the brain, usually as a result of blunt trauma. Symptoms may be those of concussion, but may persist longer. Clinical signs may range from concussion to coma, reflecting the severity of the trauma.
+ *Compression:* intracranial haemorrhage and cerebral swelling causes compression of the brain, leading to loss of consciousness and coma, depending on the extent and severity.
+ *Penetrating injury:* direct injury to the brain may result from skull fractures or when an object/implement penetrates the skull. This directly traumatises the soft tissue of the brain. Symptoms will vary depending on the site and extent of the injury.

signs and symptoms

+ Loss of consciousness (however transient)
+ Vomiting
+ Seizures
+ Slurred speech
+ Headache
+ Blurred vision
+ Drowsiness and/or disorientation

 NOTE:
These symptoms generally emerge within 24 hours of the injury, though occasionally over longer periods.

treatment

+ Call for an ambulance.
+ An unconscious patient should be assumed to have a spinal injury until proven otherwise. Therefore, full spinal precautions should be taken (see Chapter 21), after establishing a clear airway.
+ The main focus of care for the patient with a head injury is airway management and ensuring adequate ventilation and oxygenation.
+ Administer oxygen, if an oxygen unit and trained personnel are available.
+ Place the unconscious patient in the lateral position.
+ Conscious patients should rest and keep still, ensuring the head is kept above the level of the heart.

 NOTE:
Always suspect a head injury in a patient with facial injuries. DRABCD principles always take priority.

special notes

+ *Airway:* Ensure the airway is clear, but be aware that jaw clenching may be evident in severe head injury and this may make airway management difficult. Do not attempt to force the patient's jaw open or forcefully insert an oropharyngeal airway (see Chapter 23).

+ *Breathing:* Patients with head injuries may display abnormal breathing patterns. Breathing may need to be assisted with oxygen via bag and mask (if an oxygen unit and qualified personnel are present).

+ *Circulation:* Severe head injuries may cause a fast or slow heart rate. The rate should be monitored continuously.

revision

1. Complete the following sentence about consciousness.

   Consciousness ranges from full .... /responsiveness and .... in time and place to

   ...., being unaware of one's surroundings and unresponsive to ....

2. List five causes of altered consciousness/unconsciousness:

   a) _____

   b) _____

   c) _____

   d) _____

   e) _____

3. Which of the following statements about treatment for convulsive epileptic seizures is *not* true?
   a) Do not move the patient unless they are in danger.
   b) Do not put anything in the person's mouth.
   c) Time the seizure.
   d) Restrain the person if they are in danger.

4. Which of the following reasons to call an ambulance is *not* true for convulsive epileptic seizures?
   a) A seizure lasts longer than 5 minutes, or is longer than usual for an individual.
   b) The patient is a child.
   c) One seizure is followed quickly by another.
   d) The person has breathing difficulties after the seizure.

5. What are febrile convulsions?

   _____

   _____

   _____

6. Why are people with diabetes at risk of episodes of loss of consciousness and which condition is more likely to be seen by the first aider?

   _____

   _____

   _____

7. List four symptoms of hypoglycaemia:

   a) _____   b) _____

   c) _____   d) _____

continued

8. What is appropriate treatment for the conscious person with hypoglycaemia?

_____

_____

_____

9. How does treatment for hyperglycaemia differ from the above?

_____

_____

_____

10. What are the four kinds of primary brain injury?

a) _____   b) _____

c) _____   d) _____

Answers appear in Appendix 8.

wounds

learning outcomes

Perform first aid to manage the different types of wounds.

+ Describe the categories and types of wounds.
+ Detail the care requirements of wounds.
+ Demonstrate the treatment for cuts, abrasions and minor lacerations.
+ Detail the treatment for a patient with a needle stick injury.
+ Detail the treatment for a patient with an amputated body part.
+ Detail the signs and symptoms of and treatment for a patient with a crush injury.
+ Demonstrate the treatment for a patient with a foreign object embedded in the skin.
+ Detail the signs and symptoms of and treatment for a patient with an abdominal injury.
+ Detail the signs and symptoms of and treatment for a patient with a penetrating chest wound.
+ Describe the treatment for a patient with a tooth avulsion.
+ Describe the treatment for a patient with a mouth wound.
+ Detail the signs and symptoms of and treatment for a patient with an eye injury.
+ Detail the signs and symptoms of and treatment for a patient with a perforated/ruptured eardrum.

how you may be assessed

underpinning knowledge

A number of oral or written questions may be asked relating to the categories and types of wounds and the care requirements of a range of wounds – cuts, abrasions, minor lacerations, needle stick injuries, amputated body parts, crush injuries, foreign embedded objects, abdominal injuries, penetrating chest wounds, tooth avulsion, mouth wounds, eye injury and a perforated or ruptured ear drum. Examples have been included at the end of the chapter.

practical demonstration

You may be asked to demonstrate the treatment for cuts, abrasions and minor lacerations. You may be asked to demonstrate the treatment for a patient with a foreign object embedded in the skin. You may be asked to demonstrate how you would identify and treat a patient with specific wounds to their body.

scenario

You may be required to demonstrate how you would identify one or more patients suffering from one or more wounds to their bodies.

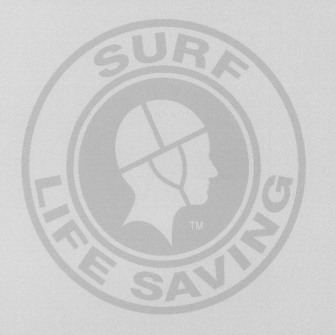

types of wounds

Wounds are injuries that affect or penetrate the skin. Wounds can be classified into various categories according to their nature and severity:

+ *minor wounds:* include cuts, abrasions, minor lacerations and avulsions
+ *puncture wounds:* include wounds caused by narrow sharp objects, such as needles and nails
+ *major wounds:* include major bleeds and penetrating injuries.

Wounds may also be classified as open or closed, depending on whether the skin is broken.

contusions

A contusion or bruise is a wound, which results from damage to the connective tissue and blood vessels under the skin causing internal bleeding and swelling. The amount of bleeding is proportional to the force involved in the injury.

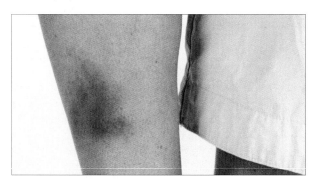

Contusion (bruise)

abrasions

Abrasions involve scraping or rubbing away of the skin. This is usually done against a hard surface, resulting in dirt and other matter becoming embedded in the wound. As such, cleaning the wound is important to avoid infection. Bleeding is usually minimal, affecting only very superficial capillaries.

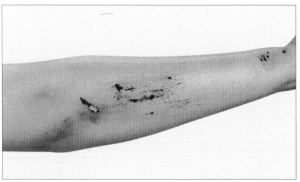

Abrasion

incisions

An incision is a smooth-edged cut that penetrates the skin and, depending on how deep it is, may affect underlying muscle, blood vessels, nerves and organs. Incisions usually bleed profusely, as they affect larger vessels. Incisions result from sharp objects, such as razors, knives and broken glass.

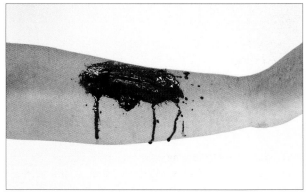

Incision

lacerations

A laceration is a cut with jagged or irregular edges that penetrates the skin. As with incisions, underlying structures (e.g. fat and muscle) may be involved depending on how deep the laceration is. Lacerations may bleed profusely, as they may affect larger vessels. Lacerations may result from sharp objects or from blunt force on skin overlying bone (e.g. skull, chin) causing it to split.

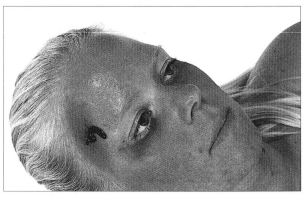

Laceration

puncture/penetrating wounds

A puncture wound results when sharp narrow objects penetrate the skin (e.g. nails, splinters, teeth). External bleeding is minimal, though internal bleeding may occur, depending on which structures are involved. Infection is a major problem with puncture wounds, as any pathogens on the penetrating object potentially lodge under the skin or deep within the body.

A penetrating wound is essentially a large puncture wound. As with puncture wounds, external bleeding is minimal if the object remains in place, though may increase on removal of the object. Internal damage may be considerable depending on the site and depth of the wound and the degree of trauma involved. Infection is also a concern.

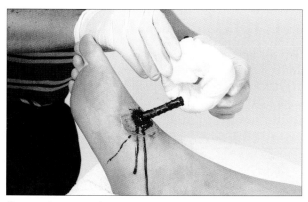

Penetrating wound

avulsions

An avulsion is the tearing away of a skin flap that may involve underlying tissues. Bleeding is usually considerable depending on the depth of the injury. A very severe avulsion with considerable force may result in amputation.

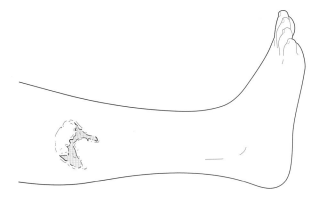

Tissue avulsion

care of wounds

All wounds need first aid to avoid infection, stop bleeding and further damage, and more severe wounds will require medical attention. While the precise treatment protocols will depend on the nature of the injury, the principles of wound treatment are to stop or minimise bleeding and protect the wound. It is beneficial to clean minor wounds (less than 2 cm in length and not deep enough to expose underlying fat) and puncture wounds, but not major wounds, which require urgent medical attention. Never wash a major wound after it has stopped bleeding, as this may disturb the wound clotting, and bleeding may start again.

Some wounds are more prone to infection due to exposure to viruses or bacteria. All infected wounds require medical attention.

The signs of infection include:

+ redness and swelling around the wound
+ pain
+ red streaks extending from the wound
+ fever

+ heat — the wound will feel hot to the patient and to the touch
+ draining pus.

cuts, abrasions and minor lacerations

treatment

+ Clean the dirty area with soap and warm water or saline solution, washing away from the wound with a gauze swab.
+ Control bleeding (see Chapter 6).
+ Cover wound, if appropriate, with a sterile, non-stick dressing, securing it firmly with a bandage or adhesive dressing.

Abrasions that contain ground-in dirt, metal or other foreign material may leave serious, unattractive scars unless promptly treated by thorough cleaning and scrubbing in hospital. This applies particularly to abrasions or cuts on the face.

Small children or patients with more extensive injuries require medical help. Do not give drinks or food, as treatment in these cases may require some form of anaesthesia. Deeper injuries or troublesome bleeding will require medical attention.

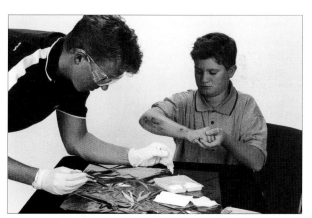

Clean abrasions with saline

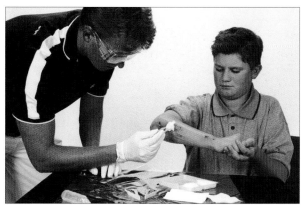

Wipe with damp gauze

NOTE:
Tetanus injections may be needed for open wounds unless the person is up to date with their immunisation schedule. For those who have been immunised already, have them consult their health care professional to see when their next vaccination is due (see Chapter 1).

needle stick injuries

Reports of needles being found on or near beaches and parks are becoming increasingly common.

Due to the risks of hepatitis B, hepatitis C and HIV infection, all needle stick injuries must be regarded as potentially serious. Even the tiniest break in the skin should be reported to the patient's doctor or the nearest major hospital. At the earliest stage, hepatitis B can be prevented by prompt injections, and the sooner they are given the better.

treatment

+ Promote bleeding at the site by squeezing wound.
+ Scrub the area gently, but thoroughly, in hot soapy water.
+ Wearing gloves and using forceps or tongs, dispose of needles in a sharps container so that the sharp end presents no further risk to anyone. Remember to take the container to the sharp, not the sharp to the container.
+ Send the patient to hospital for treatment and blood tests (see Chapter 1).
+ If the needle is still stuck in the skin, leave it in place and treat as a foreign body wound.

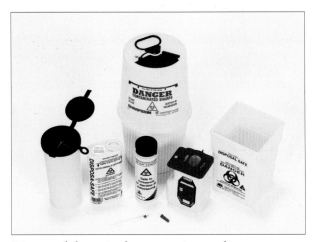

Dispose of sharps in sharps containers only

NOTE:
Take the container to the sharp, not the sharp to the container.

amputations

The severing of a body part is called an amputation. Microsurgery can often re-attach amputated parts, regaining some function, depending on the severity of the injury.

treatment

+ Call an ambulance.
+ Treat the casualty before the amputated body part.
+ Stop the bleeding from the site using a thick absorbent pad, direct pressure and an elevation sling (see Chapters 6 and 13).
+ Watch for signs of shock and treat appropriately (see Chapter 7).
+ After locating the amputated part, place the part in a clean, dry plastic bag, and seal it.
+ Place this sealed bag on top of a container (e.g. plastic bag, ice-cream container) filled with ice and water.
+ Ensure that the amputated part is sent to hospital with the patient.

NOTE:
It is important not to wash the amputated part, or let water into the plastic bag.

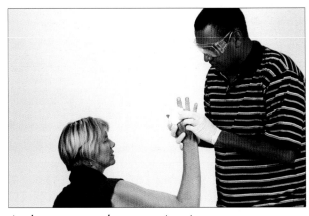

Apply pressure to the amputation site

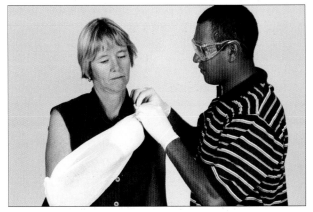

Apply a sterile dressing to the amputation site and elevate with a sling

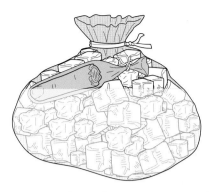

To preserve a severed part for microsurgery, seal it in a dry plastic bag and put the bag in a container on a bed of ice and water

crush injuries

Crush injuries encompass a wide range of situations, including being crushed by a car, falling masonry, mine-shaft collapse, industrial accident or by prolonged pressure due to a body part lying on an unconscious person. The common features in all crush injuries are prolonged compression involving a large muscle mass, thereby reducing circulation.

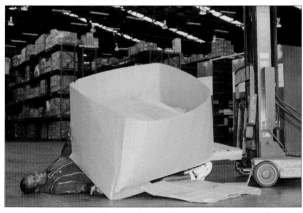

Crush injuries involve prolonged compression to a large muscle mass

signs

+ Patient trapped under or by heavy object
+ Force applied to a large area of muscle
+ Reduced circulation distal to the injury (i.e. poor skin colour, cold to touch, no palpable pulses)
+ Reduced function or inability to move the body part

symptoms

+ Shock (see Chapter 7)

treatment

+ Call an ambulance.
+ Follow DRABCD (see Chapter 3).
+ Administer oxygen, if a unit and qualified personnel are available.
+ If the body part distal to the crush site is warm, remove the crushing force immediately, if possible.

Dress any wounds, control bleeding and immobilise the injured area.
+ If there are no signs of circulation distal to the crush site, wait for the ambulance before removing the force. If in an inaccessible area, remove force and be prepared to start CPR (see Chapter 5).
+ Force applied to the head, neck, chest or abdomen should be removed immediately.
+ Treat for shock (see Chapter 7).
+ *Do not* apply a tourniquet for a crush injury.

 NOTE:
- Remove crushing force to the head, neck, chest or abdomen immediately.
- If the crushed limb is warm to touch below the crush site, remove crushing force immediately, if possible.
- If the crushed limb is cold or waxen, wait for medical help before removing force.
- Be prepared to start CPR after removing crushing force.

foreign/embedded objects

treatment

+ If an object is embedded in the skin, do not remove it, as this may cause unnecessary blood loss and further damage to the underlying tissue.
+ Place dressings (i.e. ring bandage) around the object to apply indirect pressure and stabilise the object (see Chapter 12).
+ Secure dressings in place with diagonally applied bandages (see Chapter 12).
+ Treat for shock (see Chapter 7).

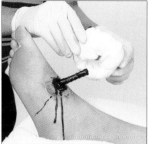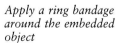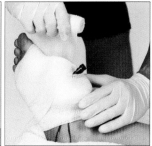

Apply a ring bandage around the embedded object   *Bandage diagonally over the padding*

abdominal injuries

The abdominal organs can be easily injured because they are covered by muscle only. Organs such as the liver, spleen and stomach can rupture and/or bleed internally and cannot be seen. These injuries can be life-threatening.

signs

- ✚ Abdominal tenderness or tightness, spasms
- ✚ History of injury to the abdominal area
- ✚ External damage or bruising
- ✚ Increasing pulse rate
- ✚ Vomiting of blood, which may look like coffee grounds
- ✚ Open abdominal wound with exposed organs
- ✚ Vomiting

symptoms

- ✚ Severe abdominal pain
- ✚ Shock
- ✚ Nausea

treatment

- ✚ Place the patient in a half-sitting position (preferably with pillows supporting their back) with their knees slightly raised using a pillow or cushion for support under the knees.
- ✚ Loosen any tight clothing.
- ✚ For open abdominal wounds, moisten a large sterile dressing, aluminium foil or plastic wrap and cover the affected site. Do *not* attempt to push any organs back into the abdomen.
- ✚ Secure the dressing with a bandage. Ensure that the bandage is loose, but secure.

NOTE:
Do not apply any pressure to the wound.

penetrating chest wounds

Penetrating chest wounds occur as a result of penetrating chest trauma, i.e. knife, bullet, fence post. Due to the relative negative pressure in the lungs prior to inspiration, air rushes into the lungs through the hole in the chest, often making a sucking sound. This can lead to a build-up of pressure in the chest cavity as all of the air does not escape out through the chest wall on exhalation.

signs

- ✚ Obvious wound to the chest wall (the penetrating object may still be in place)
- ✚ Respiratory distress
- ✚ Shallow rapid breathing
- ✚ Increased heart rate
- ✚ Frothy blood-stained fluid from the mouth
- ✚ Bubbles around the wound during expiration
- ✚ Sucking noises from the wound

symptoms

- ✚ Pain and tenderness at the site of the injury
- ✚ Pain while breathing or coughing

treatment

- ✚ Follow DRABCD (see Chapter 3).
- ✚ Call an ambulance.
- ✚ Rest and reassure the patient.
- ✚ Position the patient as upright as possible, leaning slightly towards the injured side.
- ✚ Administer oxygen, if an oxygen unit and trained personnel are available.

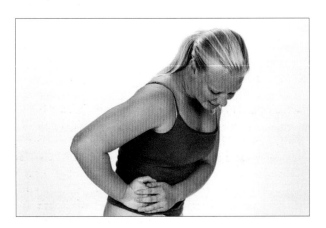

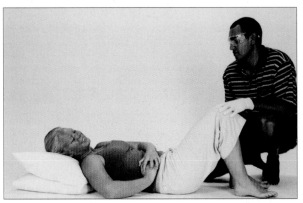

Make the person comfortable, with their hips and knees flexed, and loosen any tight clothing

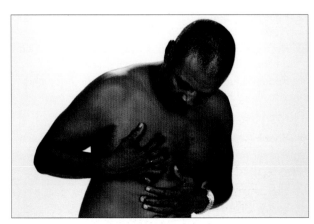

Signs of a penetrating chest wound

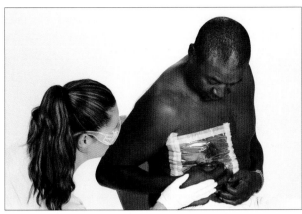

One-way valve dressing

+ Seal the wound on three sides only, with an air-tight dressing. This acts as a one-way valve, allowing air to escape, but not to enter the wound.
+ If the penetrating object is still in place, do not remove it.
+ Observe and treat the patient for signs of shock.

tooth avulsions

Tooth avulsions (when a tooth is knocked out) may affect permanent teeth in older children and adults. Assessment by a dentist is mandatory, though appropriate first aid can help save a tooth, as there is a better chance of successful re-implantation if the tooth is replaced within minutes of the accident. The longer a tooth is out of the mouth, the less chance it has of surviving.

treatment

+ Have the patient suck the tooth to clean it. Otherwise, wash it in milk but *not* in water.
+ Take the tooth firmly by the crown and try putting it back in its correct position with finger pressure and have the patient hold the tooth firmly in place until they seek dental help.
+ Have the patient bite down on a gauze pad.
+ If the tooth cannot be replaced, have the patient keep it moist by storing it between the cheek and teeth until they can reach a dentist. If the patient is too young to do this without risk of swallowing the tooth, wrap the tooth in plastic wrap.

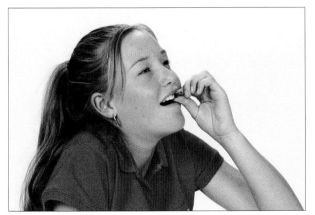

Replace the avulsed tooth and hold it firmly in place

+ Get the patient to a dentist as quickly as possible.
+ Due to the risk of choking, do not replace teeth in unconscious patients.
+ Do not let the person rinse their mouth out.

bleeding mouth

Mouth wounds are relatively common, especially in children, and often arise from biting the tongue or cheek or bleeding gums. The mouth is a highly vascular area and bleeding is usually profuse. In all cases, ensure that blood or broken teeth do not obscure the airway.

treatment

+ Do not rinse out the mouth, as this will interfere with blood clotting. Ask the person to spit out any blood pooling in their mouth.
+ Sit the conscious person up with the head leaning slightly forward (and to the side if the injury is on one side) to allow the blood to drain.
+ Place the unconscious patient on their side with the face rotated to the floor (if no head or neck injury is suspected) so the blood may drain.
+ Hold a sterile dressing over the injury and apply pressure for 10–15 minutes. Ice blocks are an effective tool for distracting patients with mouth wounds and help reduce swelling.
+ If bleeding has not subsided after 10 minutes, have the patient seek medical attention.

eye injuries

Eye injuries range from small particles or foreign bodies aggravating the surface of the eye, to major injuries, such as penetrating injuries and occluded eye. The transparent external layer of the eye over the iris (coloured circular diaphragm) and the pupil (the hole in the iris that appears black) is the cornea, while the conjunctiva covers the sclera or whites of the eye. The diameter of the iris and the pupil vary according to surrounding lighting. The lens is located behind the pupil and focuses light on the retina, which is the sensory part of the eye.

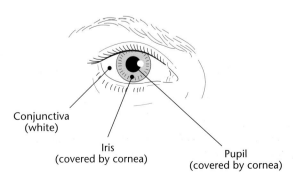

Conjunctiva (white)

Iris (covered by cornea)

Pupil (covered by cornea)

The eye

foreign body in the eye

First aid for the eye may involve removing a foreign body (sand, dirt, slithers of metal, etc).

signs

+ Pain in or behind the eye
+ Spasm of the eyelids
+ Continuous flow of tears from the eye
+ Red eye
+ Bleeding around the eye in severe cases

symptoms

+ Impaired or altered vision

treatment

+ Do not allow the patient to rub the affected eye.
+ Irrigate the eye with saline solution or use saline and an eye bath. If saline solution is unavailable have the patient cup their hands under a running tap, put their eye into the water in their hands and blink rapidly. If the foreign body fails to move easily, pad the eye and seek medical assistance.

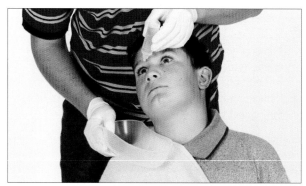

Flush the eye with sterile saline

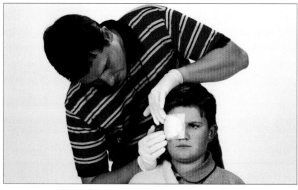

Apply a pad to the eye

+ If the foreign body is under the upper lid, pull the eyelid down over the lower lid — the lower lashes may wipe off the speck. If this method is not successful, pad the eye and refer the patient to medical assistance.
+ If irritation or discomfort persists after removal of the object, send the patient for medical advice.
+ If the foreign body is on the cornea, do not try to touch or remove it, as permanent scarring of the

cornea may result. Instead, pad the eye and refer the patient to medical care.

NOTE:
• Do not use cotton swabs to remove foreign bodies from the eye.
• Never use tweezers or similar sharp objects to remove foreign bodies from the eye.
• Do not apply pressure to an eye injury, even if bleeding.

severe eye injuries

A severe injury to the eye, such as a penetrating injury, requires urgent medical treatment.

treatment

+ Seek medical aid.
+ Reassure the patient and stay with them.
+ Even if one eye is affected, pad *both eyes*. Being deprived of sight can be very worrying to a patient, so tell the patient what you are doing and what is happening around them. If the patient becomes too anxious, remove the patch on the unaffected eye. Observe and treat the patient for shock (see Chapter 7).

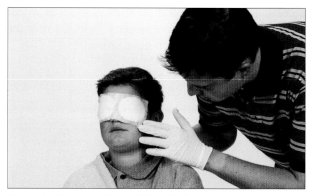

Cover both eyes with padding, if the patient can tolerate complete loss of vision

embedded object

+ If an object is embedded in the eye, leave it in place by placing padding around it and covering it for

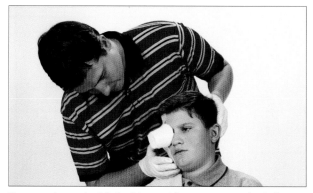

Protect the embedded object with a cup or makeshift cone and take care not to apply pressure when bandaging

protection (e.g. with a paper or polystyrene cup or makeshift cone) before bandaging. Take care to ensure no pressure is exerted on the eye or the protruding object.

swollen

+ If the eyelids are swollen after blunt trauma to the eye region, gently apply cold compresses to reduce swelling. If blood is pooling in the eye or the eye has suffered any trauma, seek urgent medical assistance.
+ Administer oxygen, if an oxygen unit and qualified personnel are available.

NOTE:
Never attempt to remove an embedded object from the eye.

perforated/ ruptured eardrum

The eardrum separates the outer ear from the middle ear (the section of the ear that amplifies sound before transmitting it to the inner ear). The eardrum can be easily injured by direct perforation by objects inserted into the ear (especially in children), by sudden pressure changes (e.g. explosion, deep-sea diving) or infection (otitis media).

signs

+ Deafness or significantly impaired hearing
+ Fluid drainage from the ear — clear, pus or blood
+ Elevated temperature, if it occurs in conjunction with an ear infection

symptoms

+ Buzzing noise in the ear
+ Pain

treatment

+ Loosely cover the ear with a sterile dressing to protect against infection.
+ Do not use any eardrops without medical advice and keep the patient's ear dry.
+ Refer the patient for medical treatment.
+ If the incident involved trauma or deep-sea diving, it may be necessary to call an ambulance. If so, continue to observe and treat the patient until medical assistance arrives.

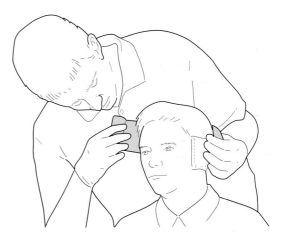

Loosely cover the ear with a sterile dressing

revision

1. What are the three categories of wounds based on their nature and severity? Give examples of each type.

    a) _____

    b) _____

    c) _____

2. Which wounds should be cleaned?

    _____

    _____

3. What should you do with an avulsed body part in the event of an amputation?

    _____

    _____

    _____

4. How do you create an open-valve dressing?

    _____

    _____

5. How should you clean and store an avulsed tooth if it cannot be replaced in a person's mouth?

    _____

    _____

    _____

6. List the signs and symptoms of a foreign body in the eye:

    a) _____   b) _____

    c) _____   d) _____

    e) _____   f) _____

7. What are the signs of a ruptured eardrum?

    a) _____

    b) _____

    c) _____

Answers appear in Appendix 8.

dressings and bandages

learning outcomes

Perform first aid using appropriate dressings and bandages.

- Describe the types and functions of dressings used in first aid and emergency care.
- Demonstrate the application of dressings for wounds and injuries.
- Describe the types and functions of bandages used in first aid and emergency care.
- Demonstrate the application of bandages for bites and injuries.

how you may be assessed

underpinning knowledge

A number of oral or written questions may be asked relating to the types and functions of dressings and bandages and the application of dressings and bandages in first aid and emergency care. Examples have been included at the end of the chapter.

practical demonstration

You may be asked to demonstrate the use of dressings on specific wounds and injuries. You may be asked to demonstrate the use of bandages on bites and injuries.

scenario

You may be required to demonstrate how to apply bandages and dressings for bites and various wounds and injuries.

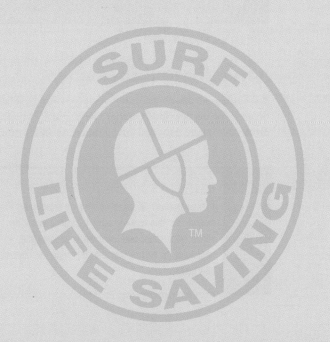

dressings

Dressings are used to soak up blood and other fluid, to assist the body in forming a clot, help reduce pain and to protect wounds from infection. Dressings come in many shapes and sizes, and are made from a range of materials.

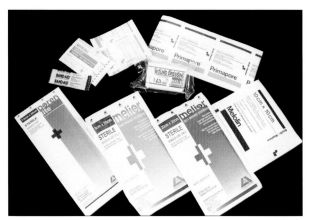

Absorbent pad dressings

non-medicated and combined dressings

Non-medicated dressings and combined dressings are used for major wounds (large or deep) where there is a lot of blood or fluid that needs to be soaked up.

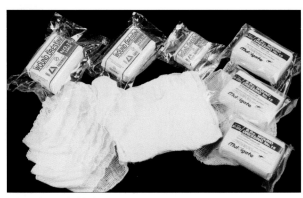

Absorbent field dressings

non-adherent dressings

Non-adherent dressings do not stick to wounds. They can be used for most wounds and are best suited to burns and abrasions where removal of bandages is likely to cause

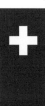

NOTE:
Dressings must be clean as they go directly on the wound. For this reason, many dressings come in sterile packaging. Take care when opening the packaging to ensure that the dressings are kept clean and sterile.

more damage to the tissue and inhibit tissue repair. Various non-adherent dressings are available for different purposes. Ensure that the dressing is applied the right way up, with the plastic film towards the wound.

adherent dressings

Adherent dressings have an absorbent dressing backed by an adhesive strip to hold the dressing in place. Adherent dressings are available in many shapes and sizes to suit different size wounds on different parts of the body. Waterproof dressings are also available, however these should be removed at least once a day to allow the wound to dry out.

bandages

Bandaging is an extremely useful first aid skill and can help to:

+ control bleeding
+ prevent swelling
+ restrict movement
+ provide support
+ protect and keep a wound clean
+ keep dressings in place.

NOTE:
Whenever applying a bandage, circulation must be checked below the bandage site — colour, temperature and pulse.

triangular bandages

A triangular bandage is a very useful addition to any first aid kit. It can be used to make a pad, a sling, a broad-fold bandage, a narrow-fold bandage or roller bandage, and it may also be used for bandaging the head, feet or hands.

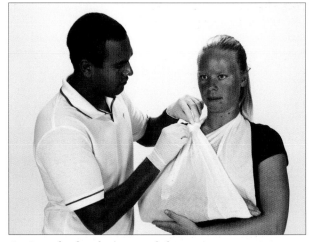

A triangular bandage around the arm

Broad bandages can be used when applying splints and for securing the arm to the body in chest injuries. They are commonly used when transporting patients who have injuries that require support and where movement needs to be limited.

Pads are used to control bleeding, cover exposed wounds or add padding to help stabilise an injury site and make the patient more comfortable.

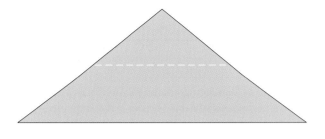

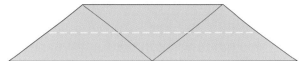

1. Place point of triangle down on base

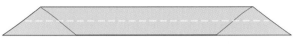

2. Fold in half to make a broad bandage

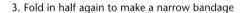

3. Fold in half again to make a narrow bandage

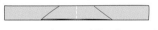

4. Bring ends to middle (do twice)

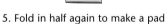

5. Fold in half again to make a pad

Folding a triangular bandage into a broad bandage, narrow bandage and pad

Narrow bandages are used to secure dressings when a roller bandage is unavailable, to secure splints to limbs and to make a collar-and-cuff sling.

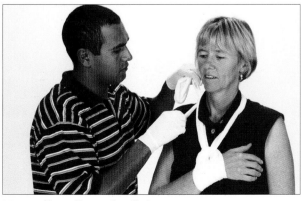

Tying off a collar and cuff sling

Reef knots

When bandaging, splinting or creating slings with triangular bandages, use a reef knot, as it will not slip and is easy to untie.

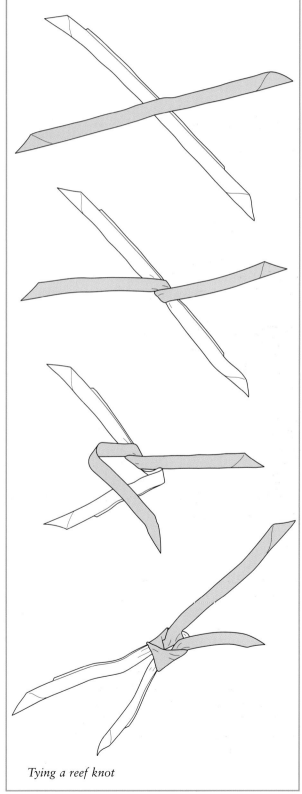

Tying a reef knot

roller bandages

Roller bandages come in various sizes and lengths, and are made from various materials. They are useful for many first aid applications, including supporting injured areas and holding dressings in place. When applying roller bandages to limbs, start distally (furthest from the trunk) and work proximally (closer to the trunk), covering one third of the previous spiral turn as you work up the limb.

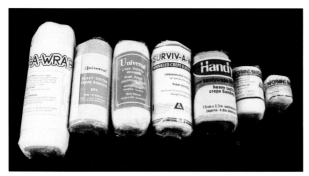

Roller bandages are available in different sizes

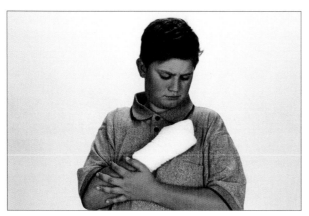

Roller bandage around the hand

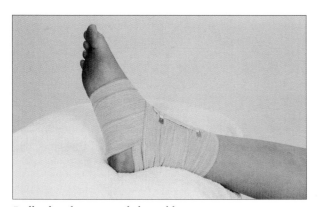

Roller bandage around the ankle

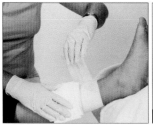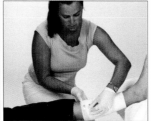

Applying compression bandaging for soft tissue injuries

NOTE:
When applying bandages, ensure that the patient is as comfortable as possible and that circulation is maintained distal to the bandage.

pressure-immobilisation bandage

This type of bandaging compresses veins and lymphatic vessels in the area of a bite or sting, reducing absorption of venom from the area, and thus delaying the onset of symptoms (until medical aid is available). It does not stop arterial blood flow (i.e. oxygen delivery) to the area.

application

+ While preparing bandages, have the patient apply direct pressure to the bitten area.
+ Firmly apply a broad crepe bandage directly over the area that has been stung or bitten and extend the bandaging up the affected limb as far as possible. A number of bandages may be required. The bandaging should be firm and the affected limb should be kept as still as possible.
+ Immobilise the limb with splints.
+ Do *not* elevate the limb or allow movement.
+ Encourage the patient to rest.
+ Do *not* remove the bandages or splints once applied.

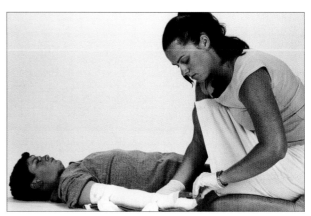

The bandaged limb should be immobilised

revision

1. List some reasons you may require dressings:

   a) _____

   b) _____

   c) _____

2. List five functions of bandages:

   a) _____

   b) _____

   c) _____

   d) _____

   e) _____

3. Which of the following statements about applying pressure-immobilisation bandaging is *not* true?
   a) Apply direct pressure to the bitten area until bandaging begins.
   b) Firmly apply a broad crepe bandage directly over the area that has been stung or bitten and extend the bandaging up the affected limb as far as possible.
   c) Immobilise the limb with splints.
   d) Elevate the limb, but do not allow movement.

Answers appear in Appendix 8.

splints and slings

learning outcomes

Perform first aid using appropriate splints and slings.

+ Describe the types of splints used in first aid and emergency care.
+ Demonstrate the application of splints for wounds and injuries.
+ Describe the types of slings used in first aid and emergency care.
+ Demonstrate the application of slings for injuries.

how you may be assessed

underpinning knowledge

A number of oral or written questions may be asked relating to the types of splints and slings used in first aid. Examples have been included at the end of the chapter.

practical demonstration

You may be asked to show how you would use a splint on a specific wound or injury. You may be asked to show how you would use a sling on a specific wound or injury.

scenario

You may be required to use splints and/or slings on one or more patients with multiple injuries.

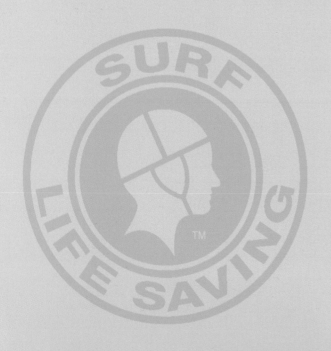

splints

Splints are used to immobilise a wounded part of the body to minimise pain, prevent movement and reduce further injury. The splint may be any material that is long, wide and firm enough to ensure the joints above and below an injury (e.g. fracture) are immobilised.

The splint must be anchored to the limb above and below the fracture site and must always be padded. It is important for the splint to fit snugly, so use extra padding around any deformity and the natural contours of the limb. Any wounds should be treated prior to splinting. Monitor the injury for swelling, pallor and numbness, which may indicate that the splint has been applied too tightly.

types of splints

Types of splints include those that are commercially available and those that are improvised (made by objects close at hand). Splints may be:

✚ soft — including bandages, towels, blankets, pillows
✚ rigid — including board or metal strips, sticks, magazines or rolled newspaper
✚ body splints — other parts of the body may be used to support and immobilise an injury, for example, strapping an injured finger to the adjacent uninjured finger, binding an injured arm to the chest or strapping the legs together.

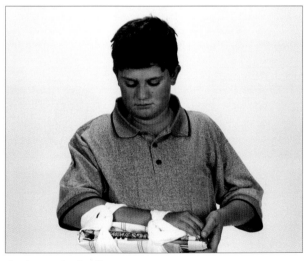

An improvised splint

NOTE:
Splints can be improvised from newspapers, magazines, wood or plastic. Clothing, towels or dressings can be used as padding.

slings

Slings provide support for hand, arm and shoulder injuries and may be used as a supplementary support for chest injuries. A number of different slings can be used depending on the type and location of the injury.

Slings can be easily made using a triangular bandage, or an improvised sling can be created using available resources such as clothing, belts or fabric. Any wounds should be treated before the sling is placed in position. Monitor circulation (colour, pulse) in the injured limb.

types of slings
arm sling

The arm sling is used for injuries to the lower arm and for some chest injuries.

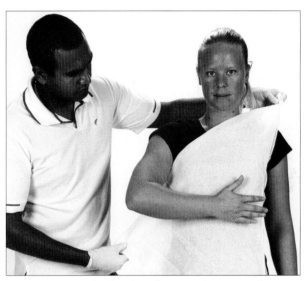

Place the triangular bandage between the arm and the chest with the apex of the triangle toward the elbow

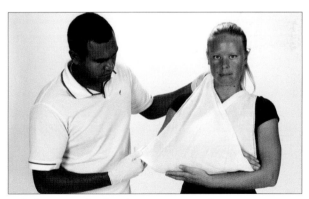

Lift the triangular bandage to support the arm

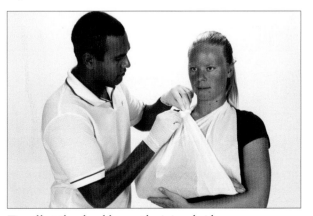

Tie off at the shoulder on the injured side

collar-and-cuff sling

The collar-and-cuff sling is used to support a fracture of the upper arm as well as elbow or shoulder injuries. This sling can also be used to elevate hand and finger injuries above the level of the heart to help reduce bleeding.

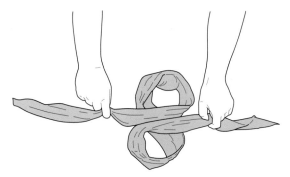

Make a clove hitch with a narrow bandage

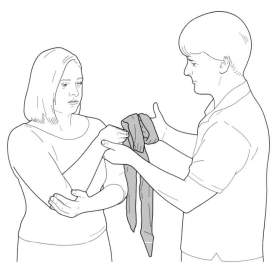

Secure the clove hitch around the wrist of the injured arm

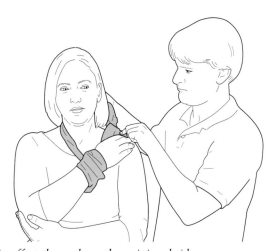

Tie off at the neck on the uninjured side

elevation sling

The elevation sling is used to support an injured shoulder, fractured ribs or a broken collarbone. It can also be used to elevate a bleeding hand or wrist.

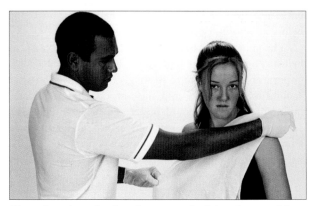

Place the triangular bandage over the injured arm with the apex of the triangle toward the elbow

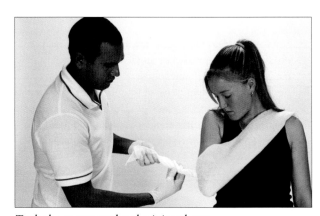

Tuck the excess under the injured arm

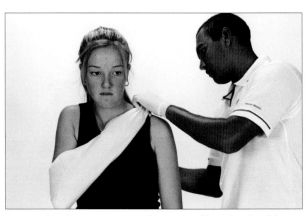

Secure the sling in position by tying off at the shoulder

Reef knots

When bandaging, splinting or creating slings with triangular bandages, use a reef knot, as it will not slip and is easy to untie (see Chapter 12 p 85).

revision

1. List the functions of a splint:

   a) _____

   b) _____

   c) _____

   d) _____

2. List examples of:

   a) Soft splints: _____

   b) Rigid splints: _____

   c) Body splints: _____

3. Which types of slings are the most commonly used?

   a) _____   b) _____   c) _____

Answers appear in Appendix 8.

poisoning

learning outcomes

Perform first aid to manage poisoning.

+ Detail the role of and contact details for the Poisons Information Centre.
+ Describe the types and examples of poisons.
+ Describe how poisoning may be prevented.
+ Detail appropriate treatment for poisoning by swallowing or inhalation.
+ Detail appropriate treatment for poisoning by skin absorption.
+ Detail appropriate treatment for a patient who has poison in the eye.
+ Detail the signs and symptoms of and treatment for a patient with suspected drug and/or substance abuse.

how you may be assessed

underpinning knowledge

A number of oral or written questions may be asked relating to the Poisons Information Centre, types of poisons, prevention of poisoning, treatment for poisoning and suspected drug or substance abuse. Examples have been included at the end of the chapter.

practical demonstration

You may be asked to show how you would contact the Poisons Information Centre and what information you would provide to them. You may be asked to demonstrate how you would treat a patient who has swallowed or inhaled a poisonous substance. You may be asked to demonstrate how you would treat a patient who has absorbed poison through the skin. You may be asked to demonstrate how you would treat a patient who has a poisonous substance in their eye. You may be asked how you would identify the signs and symptoms of, and what treatment you would use for a patient with suspected drug or substance abuse.

scenario

You may be required to treat one or more patients with poisoning.

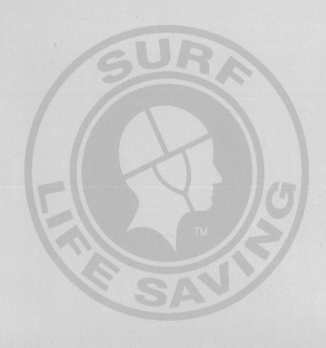

Appropriate first aid to a patient who has been poisoned can very often save their life. If the patient has collapsed or lost consciousness, call for an ambulance. If the patient is conscious and you know the poison involved, call the Poisons Information Centre (13 11 26).

Poisons Information Centre

The Poisons Information Centre is a national emergency telephone service (**13 11 26**) available 24 hours a day, 7 days a week to provide information on:

+ acute poisoning
+ venomous bites and stings
+ drug interactions.

Signs of poisoning may be apparent immediately after exposure to a substance, while others may develop over time. Never wait for symptoms to present before calling. Whenever there is any doubt, always call and check about the safety/toxicity of a product. Do not assume that a lack of safety information on product labelling means it is safe, or that the first aid information on the labelling is correct.

Legislation requires that all workplaces maintain Material Safety Data Sheets on all chemicals used within their work environment.

IMPORTANT
Always call the Poisons Information Centre for advice
— **13 11 26 (Australia-wide)** or
0800 764 766 (New Zealand)

types of poisons

Poisoning can be caused by swallowing or ingesting, breathing or inhaling, absorbing or injecting poisonous substances. Some substances may be lethal in small amounts, while others may be poisonous in large quantities or after extended exposure to the substance. Poisons are many and varied and include:

+ medication and drugs: prescription, over-the-counter, illegal, legal and herbal/homeopathic preparations
+ household cleaning products: bleach, kitchen and laundry detergents
+ insecticides and rodent poisons: sprays, baits and repellents
+ personal products: perfume/aftershave, hair dye, nail polish and nail polish remover, mouthwash, toothpaste, deodorant, cosmetics
+ garden products: fertiliser, herbicides, pesticides, potting mix
+ paints and thinners
+ petrol, kerosene
+ car products: cleaning and maintenance products
+ handyman/building products
+ pool cleaning and maintenance products
+ industrial chemicals, solvents, etc
+ bites: insects, snakes, spiders, cane toads, marine creatures (see Chapter 15)
+ plants: leaves, berries and sap from various trees and shrubs, some mushrooms.

prevention

Prevention of poisoning is always preferable to treatment. Children (and pets) are at greatest risk of poisoning because of their inquisitive nature and because they are likely to put anything in their mouths. Children can be

Poisons Information Centres

Please call **13 11 26** (24-hour line) for information and advice on emergency treatment for poisoning, bites and stings in all Australian States and Territories.

New South Wales
The Children's Hospital at Westmead
Hawkesbury Road
WESTMEAD NSW 2148
Ph: (02) 9845 3111
Victoria
Royal Children's Hospital
Flemington Road
PARKVILLE VIC 3052
Ph: (03) 9345 5680
Queensland
Royal Children's Hospital
Herston Road
HERSTON QLD 4029
Ph: 13 11 26

South Australia
Ph: 13 11 26
Western Australia
Sir Charles Gairdner Hospital
Hospital Avenue
NEDLANDS WA 6009
Ph: 13 11 26
Tasmania
Ph: 13 11 26
Northern Territory
Ph: 13 11 26
Australian Capital Territory
The Canberra Hospital
GARRAN ACT 2605
Ph: (02) 6244 3333

New Zealand
Ph: 0800 764 766
[0800 POISON]

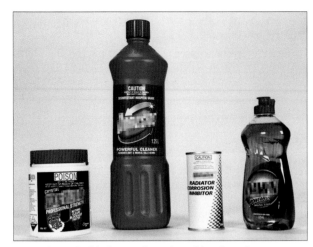

Many household chemicals such as bleaches, detergents and car maintenance products can be poisonous

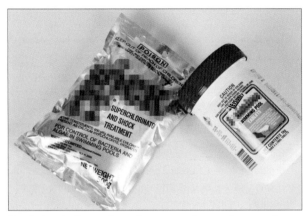

Pool chemicals can be poisonous and must be stored securely

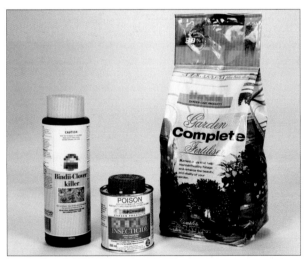

Many gardening products are poisonous

particularly vulnerable when routines and practices are relaxed, such as when moving house, when shopping bags are in the car or at home before the shopping is put away, or when visitors' bags are lying around. The following list suggests ways of minimising exposure to poisons, ensuring they are stored safely away from children.

✚ Keep the Poisons Information Centre's number by the phone — 13 11 26.
✚ Store all medicines, cleaners and chemicals out of reach and out of sight of children (i.e. more than 1.5 m off the floor or in cupboards with locks or child-resistant latches). When using them, ensure they are always out of reach of children and never left unattended.
✚ Never use other people's medication. 'Medicine' is used in the broadest possible term and includes pharmaceuticals, dietary supplements, herbals and vitamins (e.g. iron overdose from unintentional ingestion of iron supplements can be lethal in children).
✚ Refer to medicine as such in front of children, and never refer to medicines as sweets or lollies.
✚ Always read the label before taking medicine and never use in the dark.
✚ Do not take medicine in front of children as they may mimic your behaviour, and always put medication away immediately after use.
✚ Regularly review the medicines you have and take old and unwanted medicines to a pharmacy for disposal.
✚ Always try to buy chemicals/cleaners and medicines in child-proof packaging. Periodically ensure that the child-resistant mechanism is working.
✚ Educate children from an early age about the dangers of taking medication that is not for them, or other poisons.
✚ Do not transfer poisons into unlabelled containers and never transfer into food or drink containers.
✚ Remember to rinse out bottles of liquid medication or cleaners in water before disposing of, or recycling, containers.
✚ Do not leave paint brushes/rollers to soak in mineral turpentine.
✚ Always ensure proper safety instructions are followed before using paints, cleaning products and chemicals. Only use in well-ventilated areas.
✚ Become familiar with noxious plants in your garden and have them removed. Become familiar with noxious plants in your area as well. Never eat anything from the garden, unless you know it is safe and educate your children to do the same.
✚ Use child- and pet-friendly snail pellets in the garden, if necessary.

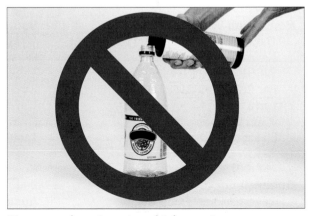

Never transfer poisons into drink containers

treatment

In all cases of poisoning, check and monitor the patient's airway, breathing and circulation. If the patient has collapsed or lost consciousness, always call an ambulance, be prepared to perform EAR or CPR (see Chapters 4, 5), administer first aid as described below and call the Poisons Information Centre to find out what else should be done.

Where poisons can be identified and the patient is conscious, do not rely on the label for first aid advice, as this may be inappropriate or out of date. Call the Poisons Information Centre.

poisoning by swallowing

+ Follow DRABCD (see Chapter 3).
+ Do not induce vomiting, unless instructed by the Poisons Information Centre, hospital emergency department, ambulance service or medical practitioner. A strong poison that burns the throat on the way down will cause further damage if vomited back up.
+ If instructed to induce vomiting, have the patient place their fingers in their throat to trigger the gag reflex.
+ If possible, identify the poison. If it is not possible or safe to take the container of poison to the phone, write down what it is.
+ Call the Poisons Information Centre on 13 11 26.
+ If the patient vomits, maintain a clear airway. Wear gloves before cleaning out the mouth to protect yourself from exposure to the poison. If you don't know what type of poison has been ingested, save some of the vomitus for analysis.
+ Reassure the patient and keep them comfortable. Roll them into the lateral position until medical help arrives.
+ Remove any clothing on which the poison has been spilled and, if skin has come into contact with the poison, flush the area with water.

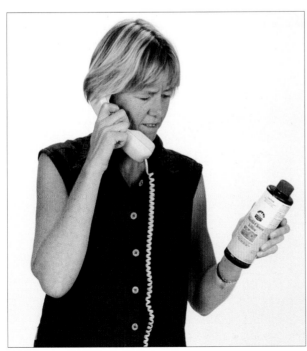

Take the container of poison to the phone and call the Poisons Information Centre, if it is safe to do so

NOTE:
• Do *not* give an unconscious person anything by mouth.
• Do *not* induce vomiting unless you are told to do so by the Poisons Information Centre or a doctor.

poisoning by inhalation

+ Follow DRABCD (see Chapter 3).
+ If it is safe to rescue the person, get them to fresh air as quickly as possible. Hold a wet cloth over your nose and mouth to protect yourself from the fumes. Call for emergency help if it is too dangerous to rescue the person.

NOTE:
Never rescue someone without notifying other people first.

+ Open windows and doors to remove the fumes, if it is safe to do so.
+ Check the patient's airway, breathing and circulation. If necessary, perform EAR or CPR (see Chapters 4, 5).
+ If you can identify the poison, take the container to the phone, or if not safe to do so, write down the name of the poison and call the Poisons Information Centre on 13 11 26.
+ If necessary, apply first aid for other conditions or reactions to the poisoning (e.g. skin burns, eye irritations/burns).
+ If the patient vomits, protect the airway.
+ Even if the patient seems unaffected, call for medical aid.

poisoning by skin absorption

+ Follow DRABCD (see Chapter 3).
+ Wearing gloves, remove any contaminated clothing, being very careful to avoid further skin contact with the poison.
+ Hold skin under running water until medical personnel arrive, or for at least 20 minutes.
+ Gently wash the area with soap and water, taking care to rinse well.
+ If you can identify the poison, take the container to the phone, or if not safe to do so, write down the name of the poison and call the Poisons Information Centre on 13 11 26.

poison in the eye

+ Holding the eyelid open, flood the eye with clean water until medical personnel arrive. This can be done with a cup or similar vessel or under a gently running tap (see Chapter 11).
+ If you can identify the poison, take the container to the phone, or if that is not safe, write down the name of the poison and call the Poisons Information Centre on 13 11 26.

IMPORTANT
- Do *not* try to neutralise the poison with any substance, unless you are told to do so by the Poisons Information Centre or a doctor.
- Do *not* use any 'cure-all' antidote.
- Do *not* wait for symptoms to develop if you suspect that someone has been poisoned.

drug and substance abuse

The signs of substance abuse (see Chapter 19 for more information on specific drugs) depend on the drug or substance taken, though signs and symptoms may include the following.

signs

- Altered level of consciousness
- Abnormal pupil size or response — pupils may be dilated, pinpoint (as for heroin overdose) or unresponsive to light (i.e. do not get smaller when a light is shone in the eye)
- Irrational behaviour — delusional, paranoid, violent, aggressive
- Sweating, or absence of sweating if the person presents with an overheating disorder (e.g. at a night club or rave)
- Evidence of a suicide note
- Evidence of empty bottles or containers near the patient
- Heavy smell of alcohol on a person's breath
- Seizures

symptoms

- Agitation
- Unsteady on feet or staggering walk

- Tremor
- Difficulty breathing — may be laboured, rapid or shallow and decreased (respiratory depression).

treatment

- Call an ambulance.
- Follow DRABCD (see Chapter 3).
- Treat as for poisoning after calling for medical assistance.
- If the patient is unconscious, turn them on their side and care for the airway, breathing and circulation.
- If the person is conscious, try to stop them taking any more drugs/substances without placing yourself in any danger.
- Loosen any tight clothing around the neck and waist.
- If the patient has a seizure, treat for epilepsy (see Chapter 10).
- If the patient presents with hyperthermia, treat for same (see Chapter 16).
- The very anxious and panicky patient may be 'talked down' by gaining their trust and attention, gently moving them (without restraining them) to a quiet place to reduce sensory overload (i.e. less noise, movement and light) talking to them calmly, reassuring them that the symptoms will subside in time. Treat for hyperventilation, as necessary (see Chapter 8).
- Try and find out what substance or drug has been taken, so you can inform paramedics when they arrive.

NOTE:
- Do not place yourself in any danger. Some drugs and substances may cause irrational and aggressive behaviour.
- Do not try to reason with the patient or expect them to behave rationally.

revision

1. What does the Poisons Information Centre provide information on?

   a) _____   b) _____   c) _____

2. List five personal products that may be poisonous:

   a) _____   b) _____   c) _____

   d) _____   e) _____

3. List the ways in which poisoning may occur:

   a) _____   b) _____

   c) _____   d) _____

4. Which of the following statements about poisoning is *not* true?
   a) Inducing vomiting is appropriate treatment for most types of poisoning by mouth.
   b) Do not try to neutralise a poison with any substance, unless you are told to do so by the Poisons Information Centre or a doctor.
   c) Do not wait for symptoms to develop if you suspect that someone has been poisoned.
   d) None of the above.

5. List five signs of drug or substance abuse:

   a) _____   b) _____

   c) _____   d) _____

   e) _____

Answers appear in Appendix 8.

bites and stings

learning outcomes

Perform first aid to manage bites and stings.

+ Describe how to identify bites and stings.
+ Detail the key principles of treatment for bites and stings.
+ Describe the general treatment principles for envenomation.
+ Describe how to identify marine bites and stings.
+ Detail the signs and symptoms of and treatment for a patient with a marine bite/sting and envenomation.
+ Detail the signs and symptoms of and treatment for a patent with a terrestrial bite/sting and envenomation.

how you may be assessed

underpinning knowledge

A number of oral or written questions may be asked relating to the identification of bites and stings, treatment of bites and stings, envenomation, marine bites and stings, and terrestrial bites and stings. Examples have been included at the end of the chapter.

practical demonstration

You may be asked to identify marine and terrestrial bites and stings and explain the key principles of treatment. You may be asked to demonstrate how you would treat bites and stings. You may be asked to demonstrate the general treatment for envenomation.

scenario

You may be required to treat one or more patients who have suffered bites and stings either in the surf, on the beach, around the home or in the garden.

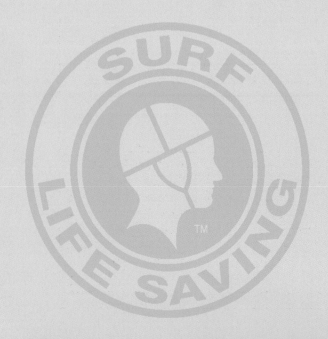

identifying bites and stings

There are many animals and insects in Australia that can deliver stings and bites capable of affecting humans. The effects can range from simple rashes and slight stinging sensations to extreme pain, respiratory depression, cardiac arrest and death.

Identification of the bite or sting may be obvious if the bite was observed and the animal seen. Envenomation should be suspected in this scenario. Similarly, some types of bites are more obvious than others, for example the twin puncture marks of a snake bite, a bee sting with the venom sac still in place or an attached tick. Most bites and stings are associated with redness, swelling or pain at the site, though symptoms depend on the patient's sensitivity and the creature involved.

In cases where no bite was noticed (i.e. no immediate pain at the site or the person was asleep or not looking) and no animal seen, the bite may be harder to identify. Obviously, in this scenario, any emerging symptoms may not immediately be attributed to envenomation.

key principles of treatment

+ Follow DRABCD (See Chapter 3).
+ Remain with the patient and send others for help.
+ Resuscitate the patient, if necessary (see Chapters 4, 5).
+ Treat and reassure the patient.

general treatment principles for envenomation

First aid for envenomation involves:

+ preventing further envenomation
+ pain management
+ resuscitation, as necessary.

pain management
cold treatment

For localised skin pain from bites (red-back spider, centipedes, etc) and all jellyfish stings.

+ Apply a cold pack (wrapped in cloth) or ice (wrapped in polythene bag) to the site for 5–15 minutes.
+ If pain persists, reapply the ice/cold pack for another 5–15 minutes.
+ Send for medical aid if cold fails to relieve pain or if other symptoms develop.

If a sting covers a large area, and particularly if the patient is cold or wet, using cold therapy over a large area may cause hypothermia. In these cases, 'ice massage' is recommended.

+ Tear the top 1–2 cm off an 'icy-cup' (frozen water in a cardboard cup) or hold a small block of ice with a glove or cloth. Rub the ice over the affected area.
+ Keep the rest of the patient's body warm with blankets or clothing.
+ Call an ambulance if there is unremitting skin pain, generalised pain or if other symptoms develop.

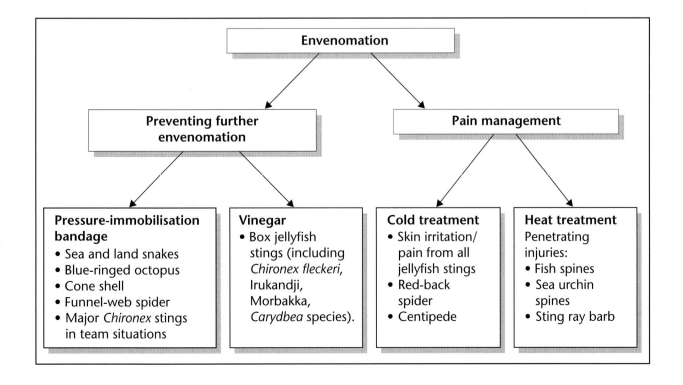

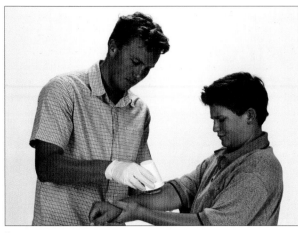

Ice massage

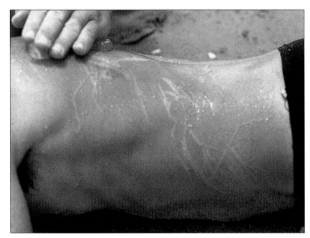

Ice massage for jellyfish stings

heat treatment

Heat stops pain in the majority of penetrating spine injuries from venomous fish (e.g. stonefish, stingray, puffer fish, lion fish, etc) and sea urchins (echinoderms).

➕ Place the affected limb in water as hot as can be tolerated (about 43ºC), after first checking the temperature, or having the patient check it themselves with an unaffected limb, to avoid scalds.
➕ Top up with more hot water as necessary, testing the temperature each time.

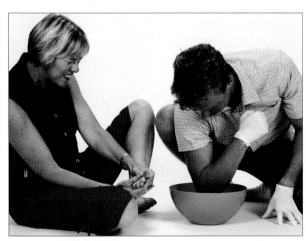

Always check the water temperature to avoid scalds

➕ If heat fails to relieve the patient's pain, or other symptoms develop, send for medical aid.
➕ Advise patient to obtain tetanus vaccination, if necessary.

preventing further envenomation

vinegar

Vinegar used for a minimum of 30 seconds prevents further stinging from tentacles that may remain on the skin after a *Chironex* box jellyfish sting. Tentacles then do not have to be removed. Vinegar may prevent further discharge of stinging cells after stings from Irukandji, Morbakka or *Carybdea* jellyfish. Vinegar does not reduce pain and does not reverse the effects of venom already injected. Vinegar should not be used on other jellyfish stings.

➕ Encourage the patient to keep the stung area still, as movement quickens absorption of the injected venom.
➕ Minor stings: apply cold packs to stung area.
➕ Major stings: CPR, if necessary, then after applying vinegar, in a team situation or if time is available, apply pressure-immobilisation bandaging (see Chapter 12).
➕ Send for medical assistance.

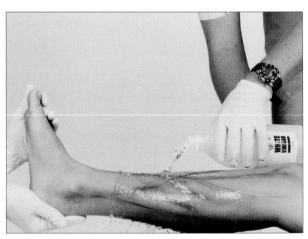

Dousing with vinegar prevents further stinging from Chironex *and other box jellyfish tentacles*

pressure-immobilisation bandage

This technique delays absorption of venom from the affected area, thereby delaying the onset of symptoms. Pressure-immobilisation bandaging (see Chapter 12) is appropriate for bites from all sea and land snakes, cone shells, funnel-web spiders and the blue-ringed octopus. In a team situation, if time permits, pressure-immobilisation bandaging should be applied to major *Chironex* box jellyfish stings.

➕ Send for medical assistance.
➕ Apply pressure bandaging directly over the affected area extending up the limb as far as possible (see Chapter 12).
➕ Immobilise the limb with splints (see Chapter 13).
➕ Do *not* elevate the limb or allow movement.
➕ Encourage the patient to rest.
➕ Continue to monitor airway, breathing and circulation.

how to identify marine bites and stings

The correct identification of marine bites and stings will dictate the treatment necessary. The following flow charts are designed to assist first aiders to identify a marine bite/sting and follow appropriate treatment specific to the type of envenomation. Identification and management of jellyfish stings are presented separately. These charts are based on material from the Australian Resuscitation Council.

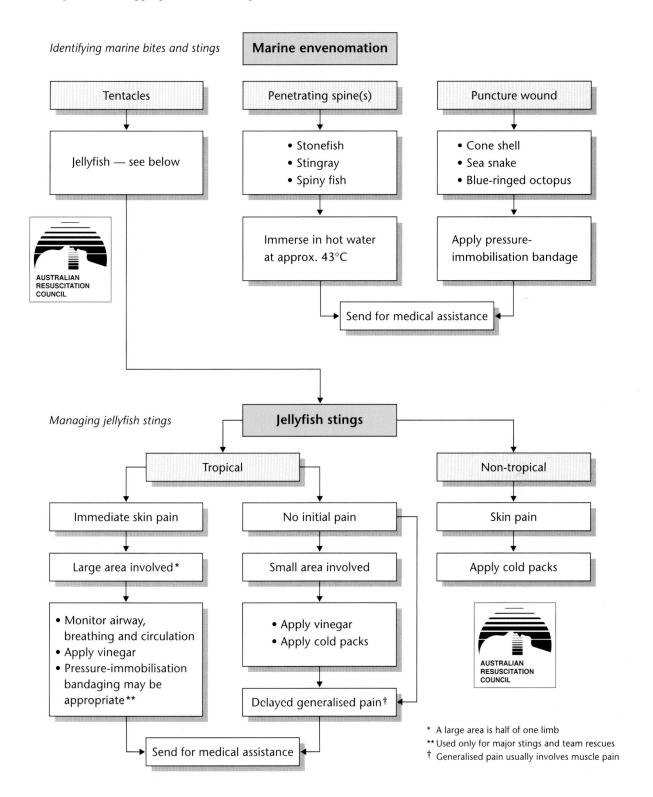

Identifying marine bites and stings

Marine envenomation

Tentacles	Penetrating spine(s)	Puncture wound
Jellyfish — see below	• Stonefish • Stingray • Spiny fish	• Cone shell • Sea snake • Blue-ringed octopus
	Immerse in hot water at approx. 43°C	Apply pressure-immobilisation bandage

Send for medical assistance

AUSTRALIAN RESUSCITATION COUNCIL

Managing jellyfish stings

Jellyfish stings

Tropical — Non-tropical

Immediate skin pain	No initial pain	Skin pain
Large area involved*	Small area involved	Apply cold packs
• Monitor airway, breathing and circulation • Apply vinegar • Pressure-immobilisation bandaging may be appropriate**	• Apply vinegar • Apply cold packs	
	Delayed generalised pain†	

Send for medical assistance

AUSTRALIAN RESUSCITATION COUNCIL

 * A large area is half of one limb
** Used only for major stings and team rescues
 † Generalised pain usually involves muscle pain

marine bites/ stings and envenomation

Australia's beach culture and easy access to the marine environment means that people regularly come in contact with venomous marine creatures. Harmless stings by jellyfish are common and are easily treated. Fortunately, fatal bites and stings are less common, but visitors to the coast should ensure that they obey warning signs and take notice of advice given by lifesavers.

physalia — 'bluebottle'

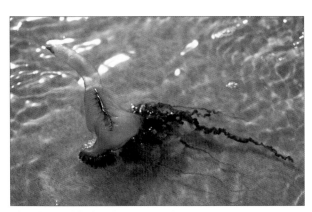

Physalia *or bluebottle*

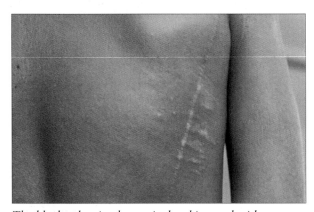

The bluebottle sting has a single white weal with 'beading'

Common names: Bluebottle, Portuguese man-o'-war, Pacific man-o'-war.
Distribution: Australia-wide and in most warm oceans worldwide.
Size and appearance: Air-filled sac up to 10 cm in length, usually with a single, long blue tentacle hanging underneath. This may contract to a few centimetres, or extend to over 1 m in length.

signs and symptoms

+ Usually a single raised white weal with prominent 'beading' effect; multiple weals may occur with mass stinging
+ Burning skin pain
+ Occasionally, pain on breathing, back pain, sweating, anxiety and nausea; often these symptoms are caused by stings from the larger *Physalia* (Pacific man-o'-war) with multiple tentacles

treatment

+ Wash off remaining tentacles with sea water, or pick them off with the fingers (the pads of the fingers are thick-skinned and only a harmless prickling may be felt). Carefully wash your hands afterwards to prevent self-stings.
+ Apply cold packs or ice, as described under pain management (p. 99).

cyanea — 'hair jellyfish'

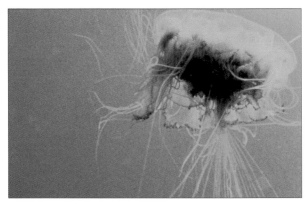

Cyanea *or hair jellyfish*

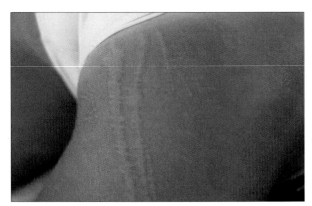

The Cyanea sting has red zigzag lines or raised white welts

Common names: Hair jellyfish, snotty.
Distribution: Worldwide.
Size and appearance: Large flat bell 4–30 cm in diameter with a large 'mop' of fine, hair-like tentacles 5–50 cm long, hanging underneath. The 'bell' top is usually white, but with yellow or brown colouring under the bell.

signs and symptoms

+ Red zigzag lines or irregular raised white welts surrounded by a red flush
+ Usually minor skin burning; occasionally more severe skin pain

treatment

+ Wash with sea water.
+ Apply a cold pack or ice, as described under pain management (p. 99).

catostylus — 'blubber'

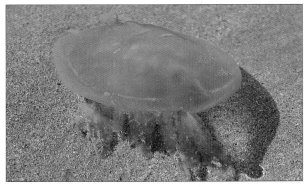

The Catostylus *or blubber*

Distribution: Worldwide.

Size and appearance: Mushroom-shaped bell 3–5 cm in diameter. No tentacles, but eight 'fronds' or 'frills' hanging underneath.

signs and symptoms

✚ Minor skin irritation only

treatment

✚ Apply a cold pack or ice, as described under pain management (p. 00).

morbakka — 'fire jelly'

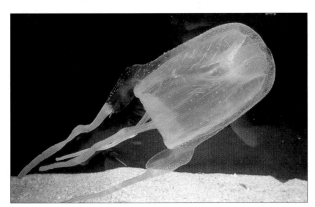

The Morbakka

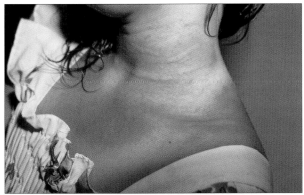

The Morbakka sting has long swollen welts with flaring of the skin

Common names: Fire jelly, *Tamoya*, Moreton Bay stinger.

Distribution: Northern Australian waters — reaching as far south as Sydney at times.

Size and appearance: Large transparent box-shaped jellyfish with one tentacle in each corner. The bell is 6–18 cm in height and has thick, ribbon-shaped tentacles up to 1 m long.

signs and symptoms

✚ Burning, itchy pain at sting site
✚ Wide, raised pink weals with surrounding bright red skin flare
✚ Occasionally, mild symptoms similar to the Irukandji syndrome

treatment

✚ Douse the sting area with vinegar for 30 seconds.
✚ Apply cold packs or ice, as described under pain management (p. 99).
✚ Refer to medical aid for further treatment.

carybdea (rastoni/xamachana) — 'jimble'

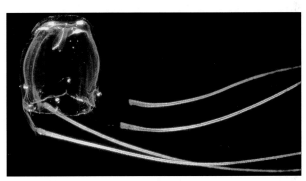

The jimble

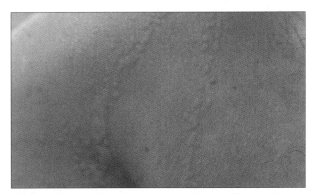

The jimble sting has thin white weals with flaring of surrounding skin

Distribution: Australia-wide — common in South Australia and Western Australia, but also occurs in New South Wales and Victoria.

Size and appearance: Transparent box-shaped bell 1.5–3 cm in diameter. Four tentacles, one in each corner, 5–30 cm long.

signs and symptoms

✚ Thin, raised white weals surrounded by bright red flare
✚ Weals are itchy
✚ Occasionally, severe local skin pain

treatment

+ Douse the sting area with vinegar for 30 seconds.
+ Apply cold packs or ice, as described under pain management (p. 99).

chironex fleckeri box jellyfish

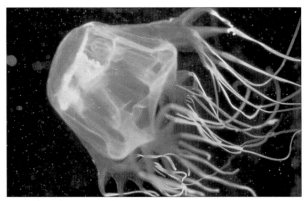

The Chironex fleckeri *box jellyfish*

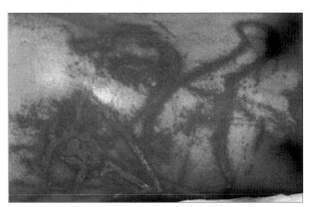

The sting of the Chironex *looks like whip marks or burns*

Common names: Box jellyfish, *Chironex fleckeri*, quaddie (named after a similar species around the Cairns area, which is not as large, nor as lethal).

Distribution: Shallow, tropical Australian waters north of Agnes Water, Queensland, all Northern Territory waters, and Western Australia north of Exmouth. This is a coastal jellyfish and it is not found offshore, although it does occur on coastal islands.

Size and appearance: Box-shaped bell up to 30 cm in diameter. Up to 15 ribbon-like tentacles arise from each of the four corners. These may be contracted to about 10 cm, or may extend up to 3 m in length.

signs and symptoms

+ Instant and severe burning skin pain
+ Sting marks look like whip marks, or burns on the skin
+ Adherent tentacles
+ A 'frosted-ladder' pattern may be visible on the skin
+ Patient may rapidly lose consciousness and stop breathing
+ Pulse may become irregular or stop

treatment

+ Follow DRABCD (see Chapter 3).
+ Remove the patient from the water and restrain, if necessary. Send others for ambulance and antivenom.

+ Administer EAR or CPR, if necessary (see Chapters 4, 5).
+ Flood the stung area with vinegar for 30 seconds minimum, as described under preventing further envenomation (p. 100).

for major stings

Major stings are those that:

+ cause breathing problems
+ cause heart irregularity
+ result in loss of consciousness or
+ cover more than half of one limb.

A pressure-immobilisation bandage (see Chapter 12) can be applied in a team situation, if time is available after attending to vinegar and DRABCD.

irukandji (*Carukia barnesi*)

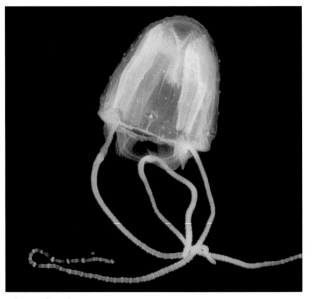

The Irukandji

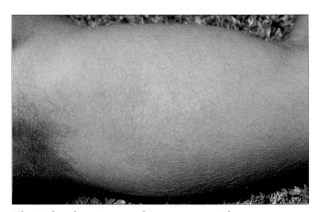

The Irukandji sting may form goose pimples or localised sweating

Distribution: Tropical Australian waters. Found in beach areas, offshore islands, out to sea, and on the Great Barrier Reef. At times they may occur in epidemic proportions.

Size and appearance: Small transparent box jellyfish, around 1.5–2.5 cm in diameter, so rarely seen.

signs and symptoms

✚ Initial minor sting; stung area may have 'goose-pimples' or localised sweating

✚ Sting is followed by a characteristic pain-free time of 5–40 minutes (usually 25–30 minutes), after which severe backache, muscle cramps, anxiety, restlessness, sweating, nausea, headache, a 'feeling of impending doom' and hypertension may develop (Irukandji syndrome)

initial treatment

✚ Apply vinegar, as described under preventing further envenomation (p. 100).

✚ Reassure the patient and make sure they rest.

treatment of established Irukandji syndrome

✚ Send for urgent medical assistance.

✚ Assess the patient's airway, breathing and circulation.

✚ Constantly reassure the patient.

blue-ringed octopus

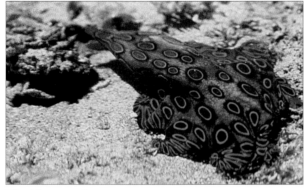

The blue-ringed octopus

Distribution: Widespread around the Australian coast (especially southern New South Wales and South Australia).

Size and appearance: May grow to 15–20 cm in diameter with its eight arms extended. Usually yellowish brown in colour, but when irritated, many small electric-blue rings appear, making it look very attractive, especially to children.

Note: Envenomation never occurs in the water, only when the creature is removed from the water and traumatised.

signs and symptoms

There is a minor, usually painless bite from a beak underneath the octopus's body. The venom is injected from the salivary glands. Symptoms rarely develop, but include:

✚ numbness of the lips and tongue may occur within minutes

✚ weakness and breathing difficulties develop rapidly

✚ in severe untreated bites, respiratory failure may lead to death.

treatment

✚ Send for immediate medical assistance.

✚ If the patient is not breathing, start EAR (see Chapter 4). Artificial ventilation will be required in hospital.

✚ Use pressure-immobilisation bandaging, as described under preventing further envenomation (p. 100; see Chapter 12).

✚ Spontaneous breathing usually returns in 3–10 hours.

 NOTE:
To date, there is no antivenom available for the blue-ringed octopus bite.

cone shell

Distribution: Cone shells can be found in shallow waters, sand flats and reefs around the tropical regions of the Australian coastline extending down the eastern and western coasts to about latitude 30ºS.

Size and appearance: Cone shells have attractive shells with distinguished colours and patterns. They grow to around 10 cm in length and have an extendable proboscis at their narrow end. This proboscis acts like a harpoon with 'barbs' (radular teeth) that inject venom.

signs and symptoms

✚ Pain (mild to severe) swelling and numbness at the site

✚ Itching and burning of skin, frequently around the ears

✚ Nausea

✚ Weakness and inco-ordination

✚ Disturbed vision, hearing and speech

✚ In severe cases, respiratory muscle paralysis may lead to death

treatment

✚ Send for immediate medical assistance.

✚ If the patient is not breathing, start EAR. Artificial ventilation may be required in hospital.

✚ Use pressure-immobilisation bandaging, as described under preventing further envenomation (p. 100; see Chapter 12).

✚ Spontaneous breathing usually returns after a few hours.

 NOTE:
To date, there is no antivenom available for the cone shell bite.

stonefish (including bullrout)

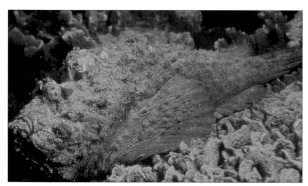

The stonefish

Distribution: Tropical Australian sea water (stonefish); fresh water (bullrout).

Size and appearance: Grow up to 20–30 cm long with a tough, warty skin that may be covered with slime. The fish is usually the colour of its surroundings (frequently dark brown) and very difficult to see. Along the back of the fish are 13 spines which, when stepped on, penetrate the skin of the patient (even through thin shoes), injecting venom.

signs and symptoms

✚ Immediate, severe pain may cause the patient to become frantic or delirious

treatment

✚ Place the stung limb in hot water, as described under pain management (p. 100).

✚ Hospital admission and antivenom may be necessary in severe cases.

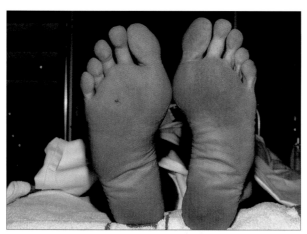

An embedded stonefish spine

stingray

Distribution: All oceans.

Appearance: A large flat fish with a whip-like tail. Burrows under the sand and can be difficult to see. When stepped on, the tail whips across driving the barb into the person's limb.

signs and symptoms

✚ The barb causes a cut or a penetrating injury — the barb may break off and remain in the wound

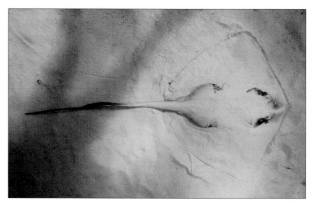

A stingray

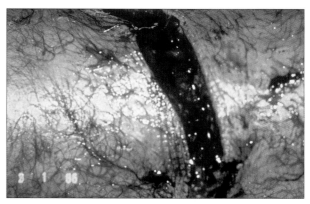

A penetrating wound from a stingray barb

✚ Bleeding
✚ Severe local pain

treatment

✚ Place the affected limb in hot water, as described under pain management (p. 100).

✚ Patients must be referred to a doctor, as the spine must be removed surgically and tetanus vaccination given.

sea snakes

Distribution: Mainly tropical Australian waters.

Size and appearance: May grow several metres long; look similar to land snakes, but have a flattened, oar-like tail; they have no gills.

signs and symptoms

✚ Relatively painless bite occasionally followed later by drowsiness, vomiting, weakness, visual disturbances, breathing problems and muscle pain

 NOTE:
Venom is not always injected when sea snakes bite, so symptoms may not develop.

treatment

✚ Apply a pressure-immobilisation bandage, as described under preventing further envenomation (p. 100; see Chapter 12).

+ Transfer the patient to hospital for assessment and possible treatment with antivenom.

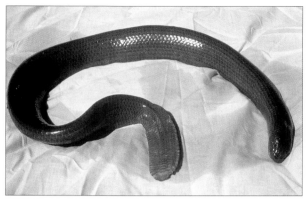

A sea snake

sea urchins

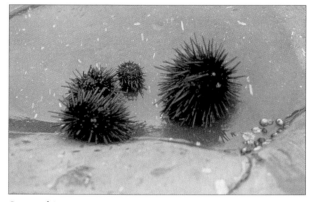

Sea urchins

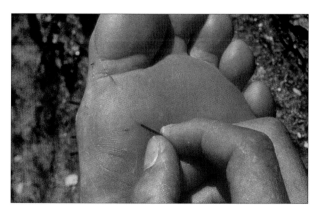

Removing a sea urchin spine

Distribution: All oceans. Often found in the cracks of rocks, so are usually not seen until the spines puncture the feet of surfers or people clambering on rocks.
Size and appearance: 'Spiky balls' of varying sizes with many long spines.

signs and symptoms

+ Painful puncture wounds; spines may break off in the wound

treatment

+ Place the affected limb in hot water, as described under pain management (p. 100).

+ Patients must be referred to a doctor, as the spine may need to be removed surgically and tetanus vaccination given.

platypus

The male platypus has a poisonous spur on the inside of each hind leg and should not be handled.

signs and symptoms

The symptoms of platypus envenomation may persist for days, even weeks and include:

+ swelling
+ severe pain
+ loss of function of the affected limb.

treatment

+ No specific treatment recommended.
+ Analgesics are required, send for medical aid.
+ Ensure that the patient's tetanus vaccination is up to date.

terrestrial bites/ stings and envenomation

spider bites

The two most venomous spiders in Australia are the:

+ *red-back spider*, found throughout Australia and often in dry, dark places around the home, garden shed and garage. Only the female is a risk to humans, as the fangs of the male spider are too small to penetrate skin.

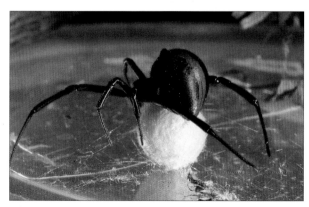

The red-back spider

+ *Sydney funnel-web spider*, whose venom can kill an adult — in fact the Sydney funnel-web spider (*Atrax robustus*) is the most venomous spider in the world. This spider is usually found within a 160 km radius of Sydney and has been recorded north to the Hunter River, south to the Shoalhaven River and westwards to Lithgow. Most bites occur in summer or early autumn, when male spiders wander around in search of a mate, or after nests are disturbed by rain, or physical damage, such as gardening. Not all bites result in envenomation, however, when dangerous quantities of venom accompany bites, envenomation is rapid and progressive, and death can occur within an hour.

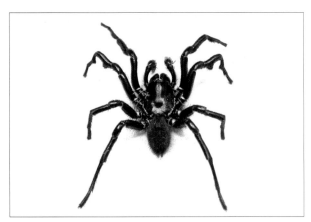

The Sydney funnel-web spider

NOTE:
Antivenom is available to treat confirmed envenomation from red-back and Sydney funnel-web spider bites.

signs and symptoms

red-back spider bite

+ Acute pain at site of bite, which progresses to involve entire limb (as most bites affect limbs)
+ Fleeting joint pains
+ Nausea, vomiting and sweating
+ Headache
+ Fever

funnel-web spider bite

+ Pain at site of bite
+ Tingling and numbness around mouth, tongue twitching
+ Secretion of saliva and sweat as well as runny eyes
+ Small hairs stand on end (piloerection)
+ Confusion progressing to coma
+ Nausea and vomiting
+ Breathing difficulty and generalised muscle twitching (including the tongue and intercostal muscles, which may cause difficulty managing the airway)
+ Increased blood pressure, pulse, and cardiac arrhythmias. Progressive hypotension (low blood pressure) develops in cases of severe envenomation

treatment

red-back spider bite

+ Follow DRABCD (see Chapter 3).
+ Rest patient and reassure them.
+ Apply an ice pack to the area, as described under pain management (p. 99).
+ Refer to medical assistance.
+ Do not use a pressure-immobilisation bandage.

funnel-web spider bite

+ Follow DRABCD (see Chapter 3).
+ Lie the patient down and reassure them.
+ Apply a pressure-immobilisation bandage, as described under preventing further envenomation (p. 100; see Chapter 12).
+ Send for urgent medical assistance.
+ Do not elevate the bitten area.
+ Antivenom is available for funnel-web spider bites.

snake bites

Australia has a large number of snakes capable of delivering a lethal bite to humans. Snake venom can cause a range of effects in humans — the most common and early life-threatening effect is muscle paralysis, which kills by causing respiratory failure. Other severe effects are serious bleeding and clotting disorders, muscle and kidney damage.

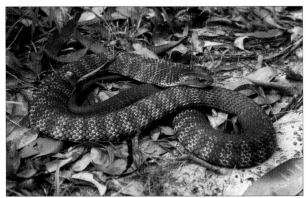

A tiger snake

signs and symptoms

Note that a snake bite may be painless and without visible marks, and that venom may not be injected in every bite (a 'dry' bite describes when a snake bites but does not inject venom). However, when treating snake bites, assume the snake is venomous and that venom was injected. The signs and symptoms of snake bites may include:

+ bite marks — paired fang marks, single mark or scratch
+ pain at the bite site
+ localised redness or bruising
+ headache
+ nausea and vomiting
+ abdominal pain
+ blurred or double vision and drooping eyelids
+ difficulty speaking, swallowing and/or breathing
+ swollen tender glands
+ limb weakness or paralysis
+ respiratory weakness or arrest.

NOTE:
Antivenom is available for all common Australian snakes.

treatment

+ Call for urgent medical assistance.
+ Follow DRABCD (see Chapter 3).
+ Reassure the patient and keep them at rest and as quiet as possible.
+ Quickly apply a pressure-immobilisation bandage, as described under preventing further envenomation (p. 100; see Chapter 12).

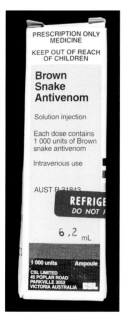

Brown snake antivenom

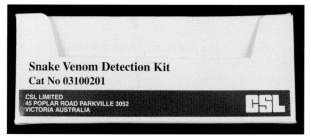

Snake venom identification kit

NOTE:
• Do not wash the affected area or discard clothing as snake identification can be obtained from the venom present.
• Never try to suck venom out.
• Do not cut the bite.
• Never apply a tourniquet for a bite.

bee and wasp stings

The majority of European honeybee (*Apis mellifera*) stings cause only localised pain (native bees do not sting). However, allergies can result in life-threatening anaphylactic shock (see Chapter 8). Allergic patients should exercise extreme caution outdoors and protect themselves by wearing long pants and long-sleeved shirts.

Hypersensitive people are encouraged to have prescribed medication readily available. More information on appropriate medication can be obtained from the family doctor.

signs and symptoms

+ Immediate local pain
+ Local redness and swelling

In an allergic person, the following may be apparent:

+ generalised itchy rash
+ facial swelling
+ wheezing and difficulty breathing
+ rapid collapse and shock.

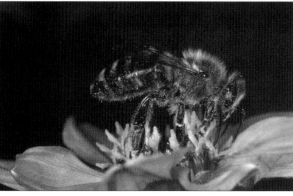

The European honeybee

treatment

+ Check the sting site for the venom sac (bee stings only) and stinger. If these are embedded in the skin, remove by any means as soon as possible. Even small delays in stinger removal will likely cause more venom to be released into the skin.
+ Apply an ice pack to the sting site or flush it with cold water to reduce swelling and relieve pain.

treatment for hypersensitive people

Life-threatening allergies may occur within minutes of a sting.

+ If prescribed medication is not available (adrenaline for anaphylaxis or steroids for systemic reactions), use pressure-immobilisation bandaging immediately (see Chapter 12).
+ Take the person to the nearest hospital emergency room or to a doctor.

tick bites

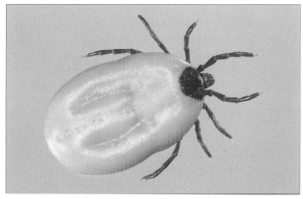

An engorged adult paralysis tick

Ticks are blood-sucking parasites encountered in the Australian bush. Ticks are found throughout Australia, though the paralysis tick (*Ixodes holocyclus*) is distributed along the eastern coastal fringe of Australia. As the name suggests, the paralysis tick contains a toxin in its saliva that causes progressive paralysis (usually localised) over a few days. Children are at greater risk of significant illness because of their smaller size. Some individuals may be allergic to tick venom and may show mild inflammatory reactions through to anaphylaxis within hours of being bitten. Ticks can carry diseases, such as tick typhus (a flu-like syndrome).

signs and symptoms

Tick bites are itchy and are often associated with inflammation and swelling around the bite, however the signs and symptoms of tick paralysis include:

+ unsteady walking
+ headache
+ flu-like symptoms
+ increasing muscular weakness in the limbs
+ tender lymph nodes
+ double or blurred vision
+ problems swallowing.

treatment

+ Remove the tick with fine curved tweezers. Press the points down onto the skin on either side of the front part of the tick (the hypostone and mouth parts), then close the points and lift or lever the tick out intact. The tick should be removed slowly allowing it to withdraw its mouth parts. Any squeezing or touching of the body may result in more toxins being injected into the patient.
+ Do not douse the tick in anything such as methylated spirits, or apply heat (heated tip of needle) as this will result in more toxin being injected into the patient.
+ The patient will need to see a doctor if all of the tick cannot be removed.
+ Check the patient carefully for other attached ticks (especially skin folds, groin, hair and hairline or throughout the hair in children).
+ If a patient is already ill, pressure-immobilisation bandaging should be used (see Chapter 12), if possible, to inhibit the movement of any toxin expressed during the removal of the tick. However, ticks are often located in areas in which it is impossible to perform this technique.
+ Medical assistance is required in severe cases of tick paralysis, which require antivenom.
+ Patients showing signs of severe allergy or paralysis need urgent medical assistance and careful monitoring.

Call an ambulance. Administer oxygen, if a unit is available and a trained operator is present, and perform EAR as necessary (see Chapter 4).

leeches

Leeches are blood-sucking parasites (annelids) typically found in dark, wet areas of bushland/forest. Leech saliva contains an anticoagulant to stop blood clotting at the bite site. The main complications with leech bites are infection at the bite site and allergic reactions.

treatment

+ Apply salt or salt water to the leech to make it detach. Untreated, a leech usually drops off after 20 minutes.
+ Wash the bite area with soap and water.
+ Apply an ice pack, if there is pain or swelling.
+ Apply pressure, if there is continued bleeding.
+ Do not pull the leech off, as the wound will bleed profusely.
+ Do not try and burn the leech off, as this is potentially hazardous to the patient.
+ Monitor for signs of allergy in people with known allergies to leeches or in those that have not been bitten before.

domestic animal bites

Domestic animal bites carry a risk of infection if the skin is broken. Children are particularly at risk of being bitten by domestic animals.

treatment

+ Minor bites or scratches should be washed with soap and water and treated with an antiseptic cream. A visit to a doctor may be wise to review the patient's tetanus immunisation status. The patient should see their GP if there are any signs of infection — redness, swelling, pus.
+ For more serious bites, stop bleeding with pressure and bandaging. The patient should see a doctor or visit a hospital emergency department, depending on the severity of the wound. Tetanus immunisation status should be checked.

revision

1. List the general treatment principles for envenomation:

    a) _____

    b) _____

    c) _____

2. List the appropriate technique to manage pain or prevent further envenomation for the following bites and stings:

    a) Snake bite: _____

    b) Stingray barb: _____

    c) Minor *Chironex* sting: _____

    d) Funnel-web spider bite: _____

    e) Red-back spider bite: _____

    f) Cone shell sting: _____

3. When is ice massage appropriate?

    _____

    _____

4. Complete the following sentences about vinegar treatment for pain management.

    Vinegar used for a minimum of .... prevents further stinging from .... that may remain on the

    skin after a .... sting. Vinegar does not reduce ....and does not reverse the effects of

    .... already injected.

5. What is the purpose of pressure-immobilisation bandaging?

    _____

    _____

6. What are the signs of a major *Chironex* box jellyfish sting?

    a) _____

    b) _____

    c) _____

    d) _____

7. List five symptoms of the Irukandji syndrome?

    a) _____

    b) _____

    c) _____

    d) _____

    e) _____

Answers appear in Appendix 8.

temperature-related illness and injury

learning outcomes

Perform first aid to manage temperature-related illnesses and injuries.

+ Describe the factors influencing cold injuries.
+ Detail the signs and symptoms of and treatment for frostbite.
+ Detail the signs and symptoms of and treatment for hypothermia.
+ Describe the types of heat illness in order of increasing severity.
+ Detail the signs and symptoms of and treatment for heat cramps.
+ Detail the signs and symptoms of and treatment for heat exhaustion.
+ Detail the signs and symptoms of and treatment for heat stroke.
+ Describe the three categories of burns and general treatment principles.
+ Detail the signs and symptoms of and treatment for ultraviolet burns.
+ Detail the signs and symptoms of and treatment for electric burns/shock.
+ Detail the signs and symptoms of and treatment for chemical burns.
+ Demonstrate appropriate treatment for a patient with a flame burn.
+ Demonstrate appropriate treatment for a patient with a scald.

how you may be assessed

underpinning knowledge

A number of oral or written questions may be asked relating to cold injuries, frostbite, hypothermia, heat injuries, heat cramps, heat exhaustion, heat stroke, burns, ultraviolet burns, electric shock and burns, chemical burns, flame burns and scalds. Examples have been included at the end of the chapter.

practical demonstration

You may be asked to show how you would recognise and treat a patient suffering from a cold-related injury. You may be asked to show how you would recognise and treat a patient suffering from a heat-related injury. You may be asked to demonstrate how you would treat a patient with a flame burn. You may be asked to demonstrate how you would treat a patient with a scald.

scenario

You may be required to treat one or more patients who have cold or heat-related injuries.

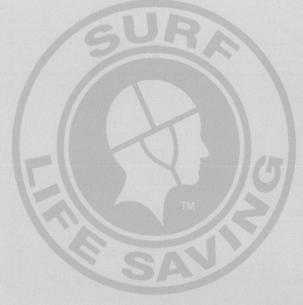

cold injury

Serious injury is possible from exposure to cold weather or water conditions. This injury may result from a decrease in peripheral tissue temperature, as in superficial or deep frostbite, or from a decrease in core body temperature, as in hypothermia.

factors influencing cold injuries

+ The environment — water or ambient temperature, wind and rain.
+ Amount of insulation (body fat or protective clothing) — lean people cool faster and women usually suffer less than men, because they have more subcutaneous fat.
+ Contact with metal or super-cooled liquids in cold weather conditions without gloves or some form of protection.
+ Exposed skin.
+ Factors affecting blood vessel dilation (vasodilation), thereby increasing heat loss (e.g. exercise, alcohol).
+ Factors affecting blood vessel constriction (vasoconstriction), thereby increasing the likelihood of cold injury (e.g. smoking).
+ Previous cold injuries.
+ Body type — slow or faster cooler.
+ Dehydration.
+ Poor food intake.
+ Diabetes and some medications affecting peripheral circulation.

In cold conditions, peripheral tissue temperature and circulation is regulated by the external ambient temperature and internal heat flow. The colder the conditions, the less peripheral circulation is permitted in an effort to prevent heat loss from the core of the body. Initially, the body's response to cold results in pain at the affected site, the skin appears red and sensation is normal. As the tissues become colder, peripheral circulation is reduced further and the skin appears pale, feels cold and may have altered sensation (e.g. pins and needles, numbness). Continuing exposure to very cold conditions will result in frostbite.

frostbite

Frostbite occurs when tissue freezes. This usually occurs in subzero temperatures, especially if there is a wind-chill factor. Mild forms of frostbite affect only the skin, and usually recover well, however, severe frostbite affects deeper tissues, including blood vessels, which deprives the area of oxygen, usually resulting in permanent damage, tissue death and gangrene. The longer the tissue remains frozen, the greater the damage. While any part of the body may be affected by frostbite, extremities such as the fingers and toes, nose and ears are particularly vulnerable, because of their large surface area to volume ratio.

signs and symptoms of superficial frostbite

+ Pins and needles in the area progressing to numbness
+ White skin that is rubbery or hard to the touch, though deeper structures feel normal
+ Loss of function
+ Swelling or blistering

signs and symptoms of deep frostbite

+ Numbness
+ White, cold, hard skin and the deeper tissues are also hard
+ Loss of function
+ Swelling or blistering

treatment

Treatment of frostbite involves rewarming the tissue. If refreezing of the tissue is a possibility before medical help arrives, do not attempt rewarming, as refreezing causes permanent damage.

+ Call for an ambulance.
+ Place the patient in a warm environment. Remove any constrictive or wet clothing and jewellery.
+ Check for signs of hypothermia and treat appropriately.
+ If the frostbite is superficial and minor, the area may be rewarmed by blowing warm air on it or by placing it against warm skin (e.g. under armpit).
+ For more serious cases when immediate medical assistance is available, wrap the affected area in sterile dressings. Take care to separate toes or fingers, if affected.
+ If immediate medical assistance is not available and there is no possibility of refreezing, rewarm the area by submersion in luke-warm water for 20–30 minutes until skin is supple and sensation has returned. Never use hot water and do not rub the area, as the ice crystals may rupture the cell membranes. If facial features are involved (e.g. nose, ears), use warm compresses over the area. This procedure will be extremely painful and tissue swelling and blistering may become apparent. Do not pierce blisters.
+ Apply a dry sterile bandage. Take care to separate toes or fingers, if affected. Protect the area from cold and movement.
+ Stay with the patient until medical help arrives. Offer the patient a warm drink (non-alcoholic), if fully alert, to warm them up and replace fluids.

NOTE:
- Do not use excessive forms of dry heat (e.g. fire, heater) to rewarm as this can burn the affected area.
- Do not give the patient alcoholic beverages and do not allow the patient to smoke, as both affect circulation.
- Do not rub the affected area.
- Do not pierce any blisters.
- Always wear gloves when handling fuel or metal in very cold conditions.

hypothermia

Hypothermia occurs when the deep body (core) temperature falls below 35°C, compromising the function of body organs. Normal body temperature is about 37°C. Hypothermia is a potentially fatal condition that requires urgent intervention to avoid cardiac and respiratory arrest.

The temperature of ocean water is always lower than body temperature, so people in the water will always lose heat. The same applies to people on land in cold conditions, especially if wet and windy.

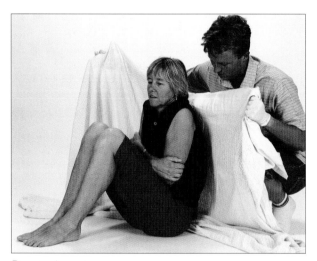

Rewarming a person

factors influencing hypothermia

+ The environment — water or ambient temperature, wind and rain.
+ Length of immersion or exposure.
+ Amount of insulation (body fat or protective clothing) — lean people cool faster.
+ Age — children cool faster than adults, though the elderly are at particular risk.
+ Activity — in water less than 24°C, exercise speeds the drop in body temperature, similarly physical exertion in cold and windy conditions will exacerbate heat loss.
+ Drugs — alcohol and marijuana speed body cooling (alcohol causes vasodilation leading to increased heat loss), inhibit the normal protective response to cold, and lessen critical judgement of cold temperatures.
+ Improper clothing and equipment.
+ Wetness.
+ Fatigue, exhaustion.
+ Dehydration.
+ Poor food intake.
+ No knowledge of hypothermia.

signs and symptoms of hypothermia

The signs and symptoms develop slowly and reflect deteriorating mental and cardiovascular function.

+ Lethargy/apathy (tiredness/'don't care' attitude)
+ Pale-to-blue, cold skin
+ Confusion, disorientation, memory loss, slurred speech
+ Drowsiness
+ Slow pulse, may be irregular

+ Slow and shallow breathing
+ Loss of muscle control, inco-ordination
+ Muscle rigidity — due to reduced peripheral circulation and increasing concentrations of lactic acid and carbon dioxide in muscle tissue
+ Uncontrollable shivering, which stops as the hypothermia worsens
+ Loss of consciousness
+ Irrational behaviour — e.g. where the person starts to take off clothing, unaware that they are cold (paradoxical undressing).

treating hypothermia

the conscious patient

The basic principles of rewarming a patient with hypothermia are to conserve and supplement the heat they have and replace the energy they are burning up to generate that heat.

Mild hypothermia can be treated on the spot with appropriate first aid, however complications are common, so referral to medical care is important. Severe hypothermia needs urgent medical attention.

+ Call an ambulance.
+ Prevent further heat loss by placing the patient in a warm environment. Remove wet clothing once the patient is sheltered from the wind, and wrap the patient's body, head and neck (not the face) in a space blanket. Cover with additional blankets.

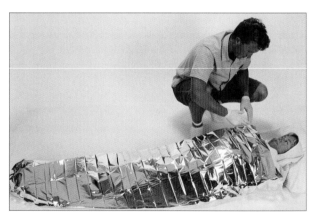

Prevent heat loss with blankets

+ Give the patient warm, sweet drinks. Do not give the patient alcohol or strong caffeine or energy drinks.
+ Curling up in a ball helps maintain heat and prevent heat loss. Body warmth from a companion lying next to the patient may help in less severe cases of hypothermia.
+ Handle the patient very gently (to help avoid cardiac dysrhythmia and cardiac arrest) and keep them lying flat, if possible.
+ Do not rub or massage the patient's limbs or try to warm the periphery in any way.
+ Stay with the patient until medical help arrives.

the unconscious patient

+ Check the patient's airway, breathing and circulation. A person with hypothermia may have very poor circulation and a slow, weak pulse, and the first aider may also be cold, so extra care is needed in assessing skin colour and movement or feeling for the carotid pulse. Perform EAR and CPR as necessary (see Chapters 4, 5).

➕ Call an ambulance immediately.
➕ Prevent further heat loss and keep the patient warm.

avoid after-drop

After-drop is the situation where the core temperature actually decreases during rewarming. This is caused by dilation of peripheral vessels in the limbs on rewarming, pumping very cold, acidic blood back into the central circulatory system, further decreasing the core body temperature. This condition can cause cardiac arrythmias and death.

Similarly, muscle activity in patients with hypothermia also pumps cold peripheral blood back to the central circulatory system, further reducing the core body temperature. A cold heart is especially prone to irregular activity and fibrillation.

To avoid after-drop do not warm the periphery of patients with hypothermia, and ensure they are handled very carefully to avoid cardiac arrhythmias (which are potentially fatal).

NOTE:
- Do not give the patient beverages containing alcohol or strong coffee.
- Do not rub or warm the extremities.
- Do not expose the patient to excessive forms of heat (e.g. fire, hot bath).
- Handle patients very carefully.

heat illness

Heat illnesses comprise three conditions in order of increasing severity — heat cramps, heat exhaustion and heat stroke. Children, the elderly and the obese are at greatest risk of heat illness, though it can affect anyone.

heat cramps

Heat cramps are painful cramps associated with strenuous activity or exertion, during which too much salt has been lost through sweating. Heat cramps are not only seen during hot weather conditions, they may be caused by excessive activity (especially in people on salt-restricted diets or certain medication) or by lack of stretching or warm-up activities prior to exertion.

signs and symptoms

The signs and symptoms of heat cramp include painful limb muscle or stomach cramps, excessive sweating, thirst, fatigue or dizziness, nausea and vomiting.

treatment

➕ Have the patient stop all activity.
➕ Rest the patient in a cool, shaded place.
➕ Loosen clothing.
➕ Give the patient small amounts of water, clear juice or sports/electrolyte drinks (which are higher in salt).
➕ Instruct the patient not to resume vigorous physical activity for a few hours.
➕ Seek medical advice if cramps do not subside in 1 hour. Patients with a heart condition and those on cardiac medication should consult their doctor if they experience heat cramps.

heat exhaustion

Patients with heat cramps may progress to heat exhaustion if symptoms are ignored or not treated properly. Heat exhaustion often happens because of excessive exposure to heat, or during strenuous exercise, such as a fun run or a triathlon, when a person fails to replace fluid loss sufficiently.

signs and symptoms

The patient will develop severe cramps, headache, poor co-ordination, stupor, confusion and poor judgement as the body temperature rises to 39°C.

treatment

➕ Have the patient stop all activity.
➕ Rest the patient in a cool, shaded place.
➕ Loosen the patient's clothing.
➕ Douse the patient with water, or place in a cool shower or bath.
➕ Cool the patient with fans, if possible, but do not allow the patient to shiver.
➕ Give the patient small amounts of water or diluted sports drink; remembering that too much too soon may cause vomiting.
➕ Seek medical advice.
➕ Anticipate that the patient may go into shock and treat appropriately (see Chapter 7).

NOTE:
- Do not underestimate the seriousness of heat-related illnesses.
- Do not give alcohol or caffeine to a person suffering from an overheating condition.
- Do not give the patient any medication to reduce a fever.

heat stroke

Heat stroke is the ultimate overheating disaster, and will occur if the earlier stages of heat exhaustion are not recognised and treated promptly. It is a progression from heat exhaustion, usually accompanied by physical collapse, in which the body temperature rises above 39°C.

signs and symptoms

The skin feels hot and dry because the sweating mechanism is 'switched off' as the body attempts to stop the loss of fluid. People become restless or aggressive, confused, disoriented and may experience seizures or lose consciousness.

Heat stroke is a life-threatening medical emergency that requires urgent medical attention. The focus of first aid is life support and reducing core body temperature by whatever means possible until medical help arrives.

Heat stroke should not be confused with sun stroke — the nausea and headache associated with too much sun exposure without a hat.

treatment

+ Treat the unconscious patient by checking the airway, breathing and circulation in the usual manner.
+ Call an ambulance immediately, as the patient will require chilled intravenous fluids and glucose. While waiting, apply the cooling methods outlined below or whatever methods are available. Do not give fluid by mouth if the patient is unconscious.
+ Apply cold packs or ice to the sides of the neck, the armpits and the groin, where large arteries are close to the surface.
+ Sometimes uncontrollable muscle twitching may occur. If so, prevent the patient from injuring themself. Do not place anything in the person's mouth and do not give the person anything to drink. If they vomit, maintain a clear airway by placing the patient on their side and removing any vomitus from the mouth (using gloves).
+ Anticipate that the patient may go into shock and treat appropriately.

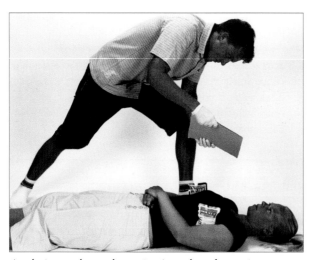

Apply ice packs to the patient's neck and armpits

prevention of heat exhaustion and heat stroke

Athletes exercising in the heat may lose 2–3 litres of fluid per hour; this must be replaced. Loss of just 5% of body fluid will impair an athlete's performance; loss of 10% of body fluid puts the athlete at great risk of heat exhaustion.

To prevent heat exhaustion and heat stroke:

+ in the 30 minutes before hard exercise in the heat, drink at least 500 mL of water
+ during the event, drink sufficient amounts of water to match loss

+ in events lasting more than an hour, it may also be necessary to use a commercial sports drink to replace carbohydrates.

burns

A burn occurs when the skin and other bodily organs come into contact with heat, radiation, electricity or chemicals long enough to cause damage. Appropriate first aid can reduce the severity of burns and the likelihood of permanent scarring.

Burns can affect many body parts other than the site of the burn. Nerves, blood vessels, bones, muscles and other areas may be involved. This is particularly so for electrocution, which may also disturb cardiac rhythm and function.

There are generally three categories of burns, depending on the depth of the injury.

 NOTE:
Do not apply any greasy substance, such as butter or creams, to the burn. This can hamper cooling of the burn area and do further damage.

superficial burns

Superficial burns (previously known as first-degree burns) involve the upper layer of skin, the epidermis. Such burns are usually a pink to reddish colour. The patient may also have signs and symptoms of mild swelling, tenderness and pain. These burns usually heal on their own with little or no signs of scarring.

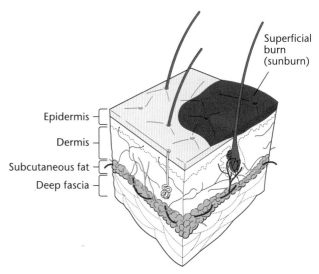

Cross-section of a superficial burn

 NOTE:
If an infant or elderly person suffers from a burn, even minor, obtain medical assistance promptly.

partial-thickness burns

Partial-thickness burns (previously known as second-degree burns) involve the first and second layers of skin — the epidermis and the dermis. The symptoms of pain and signs of swelling are similar to those of superficial burns, although the skin is usually a brighter red and blistering develops. Burns may take from 1 to 3 weeks to heal, but are considered minor if they cover no more than 15% of the total body area in adults and 10% of the body area in children. Partial-thickness burns often produce scarring and require medical attention.

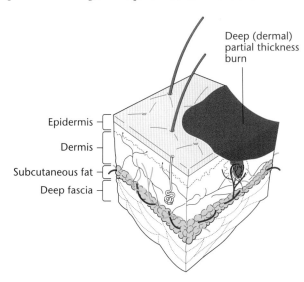

Cross-section of a partial-thickness burn

full-thickness burns

Full-thickness burns (previously known as third-degree burns) may appear charred or have white, brown or black patches. Both the dermis and epidermis are destroyed. Fatty tissue, muscle, bone and other organs may also be involved. Full-thickness burns produce deep scars that often require cosmetic or reconstructive surgery and skin grafts. Pain may or may not be present, since nerve endings, which transmit pain, may have been destroyed.

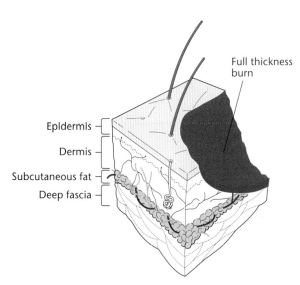

Cross-section of a full-thickness burn

severity of burns

Looking at a number of different components can help assess the severity of burns. These are:

✚ the area the burn(s) covers
✚ the depth of the burn
✚ the age and health of the person
✚ the areas the burn has damaged, e.g. a burn of the same type and size to the genitals or airway will be more severe than one to the hand.

treatment

As a general rule, burns need to be cooled. The best way of doing this is by running tap water over the area for 10–20 minutes. Medical assistance should be sought urgently for serious burns.

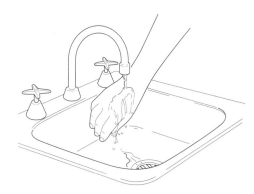

Run cold water over burns. Dress burns with burns dressings and bandages

ultraviolet burns

Sunburn is burning of the skin caused by ultraviolet rays, most commonly from sunlight. In addition to sunburn, exposure to sunlight is associated with premature skin ageing and skin cancers, including melanoma.

signs and symptoms
✚ Redness
✚ Pain
✚ Blistering
✚ Fever, chills and nausea in severe cases

treatment
✚ Have the patient rest in a cool place.
✚ Cool the sunburn with water for up to 20 minutes.
✚ Give the patient fluids by mouth.
✚ Do not prick blisters.
✚ Seek medical advice if the sunburn is extensive, especially if the patient is vomiting, dehydrated, has a severe headache, or is a child.

electrical burns/shock

Electrical burns are caused when contact is made with an electrical source or when a person is struck by lightning. Electricity is conducted through the body, usually creating an entry and exit point. Wounds may seem superficial; however, there may be greater damage to the underlying tissue and organs. Electricity may cause the heart to beat irregularly or even stop.

Where domestic electricity is involved (considered less than 1000 volts), it may be possible to separate the patient from the source by pushing the patient or power cord away with something that does not conduct electricity (e.g. wood). Always be careful to avoid water or other conducting materials in contact with the patient until the power is turned off.

If high-voltage electricity is involved (considered greater than 1 000 volts), it is not safe to be in the area as arcing can occur within 8 m of the electricity source. There is nothing that can be safely done for the patient until the power is turned off and the area declared safe, because of the extreme danger of electricity arcing through the air to earth itself through any conducting material, including you! If the patient is conscious, they should crouch down or lie down to reduce the likelihood of arcing.

If powerlines are down across a car or near it, the person should be advised to stay inside, as the rubber tyres insulate the car.

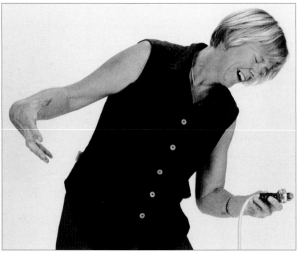

Electric shock from contact with a live source of domestic electricity

signs and symptoms

+ Unconsciousness
+ Confusion
+ Burns to skin, with (usually) an entry and an exit point
+ Irregular, weak or absent pulse

treatment

+ Follow DRABCD (see Chapter 3).
+ Turn off the electrical supply, or seek help if you are unable to disconnect the current. For example, have the

electrical company disconnect the power if powerlines are down.
+ Check the patient's airway, breathing and circulation. Perform EAR and CPR as necessary (see Chapters 4, 5).
+ Treat superficial burns with cool running water and cover with sterile non-adherent dressings.
+ Always seek medical assistance for major burns or complications.

 NOTE:
- Do not touch the patient, or any conducting material in contact with them, until the power source has been turned off.
- Never approach a patient within a high-voltage power source safety zone until the area has been declared safe.

chemical burns

Chemical burns occur when strong acids or alkalis, which are caustic, come in contact with the skin and/or the eyes. These burns commonly occur in industrial settings and may be caused by short- or long-term exposure to a chemical substance.

signs and symptoms

+ Abdominal pain
+ Blisters, rashes and burns on the skin
+ Cloudy, red or watery eyes
+ Dizziness
+ Headaches
+ Pain at the site of the injury
+ Seizures
+ Unconsciousness
+ Visual impairment
+ For airway burns — coughing, shortness of breath or difficulty breathing (e.g. wheezing)

treatment for a chemical burn to the skin

+ Rinse the exposed area with running water for at least 20 minutes.
+ Carefully remove the contaminated clothing, making sure not to touch the unaffected skin (or yourself) with the clothing.
+ Do not remove any clothing that is stuck to the skin.
+ Call for medical assistance and the Poisons Information Centre (13 11 26).

treatment for a chemical burn to the eye

✚ Rinse the eyes immediately until medical aid arrives.
✚ Call for medical assistance and advice from the Poisons Information Centre (13 11 26).

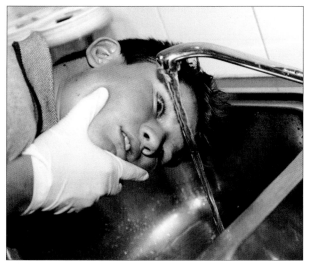

Flush the eye with copious amounts of water

flame burns

Flame burns are those associated with any naked flame. Minor burns can be adequately dealt with by first aid alone, though major burns can be life-threatening.

treatment

✚ Follow DRABCD (see Chapter 3).
✚ If a person or their clothing is on fire, stop, drop and roll. Stop the patient from running, cover them in a (non-synthetic) blanket, or similar, to smother the flames, lay them on the ground and roll them until the flames have been extinguished.
✚ Check the patient's airway, breathing and circulation. Perform EAR and CPR, as necessary (see Chapters 4, 5).

✚ Immediately treat burns with cool running water for 20 minutes. Cover with sterile non-adherent dressings.
✚ Assess the severity of the burns and call an ambulance.
✚ If the burns are severe and extensive, cover with moistened dressings or a sheet.
✚ In cases of severe burns, anticipate that the patient will go into shock and treat appropriately (see Chapter 7).

scalds

Scalds result from contact with sources of wet heat, such as boiling liquids or steam. Children are at higher risk of scalds because their skin is thinner and more prone to injury, and because they do not understand the potential danger of their exploratory actions.

treatment

✚ Quickly remove any clothing, which retains heat and may obscure other scalded areas of the body.
✚ Hold the scalded area in cool water or run under cool tap water for at least 10 minutes.
✚ Remove any tight clothing or objects, such as jewellery, which may constrict swelling.
✚ Cover the scald with sterile non-adherent dressings.
✚ Assess the severity of the scald. Minor scalds can be treated by the patient's doctor, though more severe scalds should be treated at the nearest hospital.

NOTE:
• Do not remove clothing that is stuck to the affected area.
• Do not pierce blisters.
• Do not apply any creams or lotions (especially butter or oil) to the burn as they may cause further damage and make burn classification difficult.
• Do not apply dressings that may stick to the burn and cause further damage on removal.
• Treat for shock.

revision

1. Which of the following statements about the development of cold injuries is *not* entirely true?
   a) In cold conditions, peripheral circulation is restricted to prevent core body heat loss.
   b) The body's initial response to cold results in numbness at the affected site, the skin appears blanched and sensation is normal.
   c) As the tissues become colder, peripheral circulation is reduced further and the skin appears pale, feels cold and may have altered sensation.
   d) Continuing exposure to very cold conditions will result in frostbite.

2. Complete the following sentence about frostbite.

   Mild forms of frostbite affect only the ...., and usually recover well, however, severe frostbite affects

   .... tissues, including ...., which deprives the area of oxygen, usually resulting in

   .... damage, tissue death and ....

3. Which of the following treatments for frostbite is *not* appropriate practice?
   a) Superficial frostbite may be rewarmed by blowing warm air on it or by placing it against warm skin.
   b) If immediate medical assistance is not available and there is no possibility of refreezing, rewarm the area.
   c) After rewarming apply dry sterile bandage and protect from the cold.
   d) After rewarming, encourage movement of the area to stimulate blood supply.

4. What should you *not* do to a person with hypothermia?
   a) Give them beverages containing alcohol or strong coffee.
   b) Handle them roughly.
   c) Attempt to warm or rub the extremities.
   d) All of the above.

5. List five signs and symptoms of heat cramps:

   a) _____   b) _____   c) _____

   d) _____   e) _____

6. Complete the following sentences about heat stroke.

   The skin feels hot and .... because the sweating mechanism is .... as the

   body attempts to stop the loss of .... People become restless or ...., confused,

   .... and may experience .... or lose consciousness.

7. List the three categories of burns depending on the depth of injury:

   a) _____   b) _____   c) _____

8. What are the signs and symptoms of electric shock?

   _____

   _____

9. If a person or their clothing is on fire, what should you do?

   _____

   _____

10. Which of the following statements regarding treatment for scalds is *not* entirely true?
    a) Quickly remove any clothing.
    b) Hold the scalded area in cool water or run under cool tap water for 2 minutes.
    c) Remove any tight clothing or objects, such as jewellery, which may constrict swelling.
    d) Cover the scald with sterile non-adherent dressing.

Answers appear in Appendix 8.

hard and soft tissue injuries

learning outcomes

Perform first aid to manage hard and soft tissue injuries.

- Describe the types of hard tissue injuries.
- Describe the types of fractures that may occur with hard tissue injuries.
- Detail the signs and symptoms of a fracture.
- Demonstrate the treatment for a patient who has a fracture.
- Detail the signs and symptoms of a patient who has a dislocation or subluxation.
- Demonstrate the treatment for a patient who has a dislocation or subluxation.
- Detail the signs and symptoms of the different types of soft tissue injuries.
- Demonstrate the treatment for a patient with soft tissue injuries using the RICER approach.
- Detail what a patient should avoid during the first 48–72 hours after a soft tissue injury.

how you may be assessed

underpinning knowledge

A number of oral or written questions may be asked relating to hard tissue injuries, fractures, dislocations, subluxations, soft tissue injuries, the RICER approach and immediate management of soft tissue injuries. Examples have been included at the end of the chapter.

practical demonstration

You may be asked to demonstrate how you would identify and treat a patient with a fracture. You may be asked to demonstrate how you would identify and treat a patient with a dislocation or subluxation. You may be asked how you would identify and treat a patient with soft tissue injuries using the RICER approach.

scenario

You may be required to treat one or more patients who have hard or soft tissue injuries.

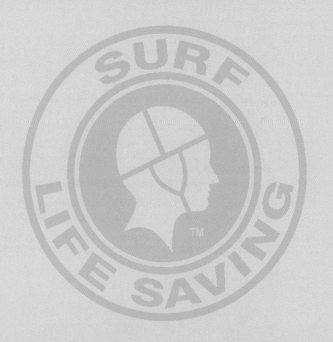

hard tissue injuries

Hard tissue injuries are those that affect bone. Hard tissue injuries include:

+ fractures, where bones are broken
+ dislocations, where bones are displaced from their usual position in joints
+ subluxations or incomplete dislocations.

When in doubt as to the severity of an injury, treat as a fracture.

fractures

types of fractures

A fracture is a break or crack in a bone. Fractures can be classified as either open or closed. An open fracture will involve an open wound. This can occur by the bone piercing the skin and soft tissue when it breaks, and the bone appearing through the skin. Alternatively, an open fracture may result from an object penetrating the skin and fracturing a bone. A closed fracture is more common and occurs when the skin remains intact (unbroken).

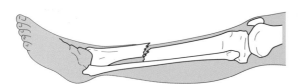

Open fracture of the tibia

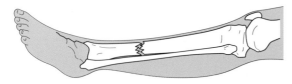

Closed fracture of the tibia

Both open and closed fractures have the potential to cause serious injury to internal body structures. While many fractures are not immediately life-threatening, fractures can cause shock and major internal and external bleeding.

signs

+ Loss of function
+ Swelling at the site, resulting from internal bleeding
+ Deformity — the affected part is changed in shape
+ Unnatural movement — the affected part can be moved too freely
+ Open fractures are self-evident with bone/s protruding from an open, bleeding wound
+ Shock (see Chapter 7)

symptoms

+ Pain and tenderness at the site
+ Feeling/sound of bone ends grating or the sound of a snap or pop at the time of injury
+ Tingling or numbness

 NOTE:
Minor fractures and dislocations, sprains and strains, are sometimes impossible to tell apart, even by skilled medical personnel. The treatment is similar.

treatment

The precise treatment of fractures depends on the location of the injury. However, these steps apply to most fractures. Treatment for specific fractures is addressed below.

+ Reassure the patient and advise them *not* to move.
+ Immobilise the injured limb in the position in which you found it.
+ If possible, leave the patient where they fell or injured themself and send for an ambulance.
+ If the patient needs to be moved, immobilise the area first.
+ Be sure to immobilise the area above and below the fracture.
+ If the fracture needs a splint it must be long enough to extend past the joint above and below the fracture site and wide enough to support the fracture site.
+ Seek medical assistance.

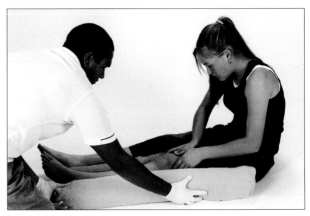

Immobilise the injured limb

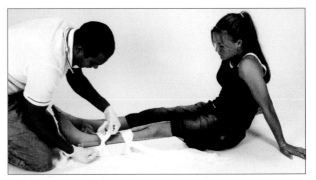

Splint the fracture with a bandage above and below the break

- Check that circulation is present beyond the fracture. If not, call for urgent medical aid.
- Control bleeding if there is an open wound and cover with sterile dressing to reduce infection.
- Check the patient for other injuries and treat appropriately.
- Apply ice packs or cold compresses, if possible, for 5–15 minutes, if pain permits. Reapply if necessary (except on open fractures, i.e. those associated with an open wound).
- Assess for shock and treat as required (see Chapter 7).

treatment for upper and lower arm fractures

- Seek medical assistance.
- Control bleeding if there is an open wound and cover with sterile dressing to reduce infection. Apply padding around protruding bone(s).
- Apply a splint from the elbow to the hand for lower arm fractures to immobilise the fracture. Elevate the fracture using an arm sling.
- If the suspected fracture involves the elbow or is very close to it, do not move the elbow. Support and immobilise the arm in the position in which you found it.
- For upper arm fractures, pad between the arm and the chest and apply a collar-and-cuff sling to immobilise the arm.
- Check that circulation is present beyond the fracture. If not, call for urgent medical aid.
- Check the patient for other injuries and treat appropriately.

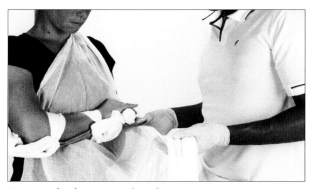

Support the fracture with a sling

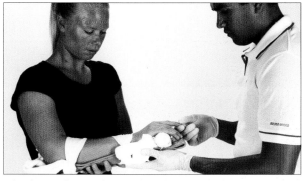

Check circulation distal to the fracture

treatment for upper and lower leg fractures

- Seek medical assistance.
- Control bleeding if there is an open wound and cover with sterile dressing to reduce infection. Apply padding around protruding bones.
- The uninjured leg may be used as a splint for upper and lower leg fractures. Pad between the legs and bring the uninjured leg to the injured leg and tie the legs together with bandages (above and below fracture, at knees and at ankles/feet) tying off on the uninjured side.
- If the ground is supporting the limb, there may be no need to splint it to the other limb.
- Check that circulation is present beyond the fracture. If not, call for urgent medical aid.
- Check the patient for other injuries and treat appropriately.

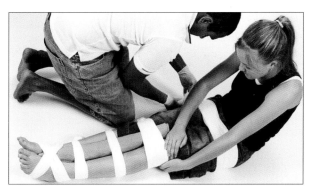

The uninjured leg can be used as a splint

treatment for hip fractures

- Seek medical assistance.
- Control bleeding if there is an open wound and cover with sterile dressing to reduce infection. Apply padding around protruding bones.
- The uninjured leg may be used as a splint for hip fractures. Pad between the legs and bring the uninjured leg to the injured leg and tie the legs together with bandages (above and below fracture, at knees and at ankles/feet) tying off on the uninjured side.
- Do not move the patient, unless they are in life-threatening danger. If they must be moved immobilise them on a spinal board or similar hard surface (see Chapter 21).
- Check that circulation is present beyond the fracture. If not, call for urgent medical aid.
- Assess for shock and treat as required (see Chapter 7).

treatment for pelvic fractures

- Seek medical assistance.
- Control bleeding if there is an open wound and cover with sterile dressing to reduce infection. Apply padding around protruding bones.
- Place the legs and feet in a comfortable position.
- Discourage the patient from urinating.

+ Assess for shock and treat as required (see Chapter 7).
+ Do not move the patient, unless they are in life-threatening danger. If they must be moved, immobilise them on a spinal board or similar hard surface (see Chapter 20).

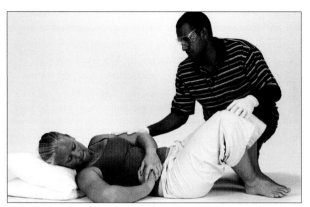

If a hip fracture is suspected, place the patient in a comfortable position, usually with the knees raised, as for abdominal injuries

fractured rib

signs

+ Short, rapid breathing
+ Local tenderness around ribs
+ Patient may support injury site with hand or arm

symptoms

+ Pain, especially when patient coughs or breathes
+ Local tenderness around ribs

treatment for the conscious patient

+ Seek medical assistance.
+ Ensure the patient is in a comfortable position. A half-sitting position resting the affected side on a pillow or cushion is ideal.
+ Encourage the patient to take shallow breaths to reduce pain.
+ Apply padding over affected ribs.
+ Place the arm on the same side as the injury over the pad.
+ Secure with broad bandages over the arm and around the body, tying them off on the non-injured side.
+ Immobilise the arm on the affected side using an appropriate sling.

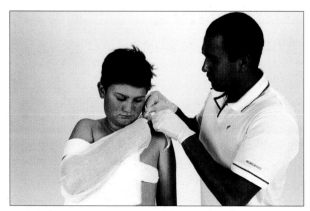

Pad and tie a broad bandage around the affected rib and immobilise the arm on the affected side using a sling

NOTE:
+ Absence of circulation constitutes a medical emergency. Seek medical aid. Some minor movement of the area may be needed to re-establish circulation.
+ Do not move the patient unless necessary and after the fracture has been immobilised.
+ Do not move a patient with an injured hip or dislocated thigh unless it is absolutely necessary.
+ Do not test the range of movement or function of a suspected broken bone.
+ Do not attempt to straighten or realign a broken bone.
+ Do not give the person anything to eat or drink.

treatment for the unconscious patient

+ Seek medical assistance.
+ Follow DRABCD (see Chapter 3).
+ Place the patient in the lateral position with the injured side down.

dislocation

A dislocation is an injury in which a bone is moved out of its normal position in relation to another bone with which it forms a joint. The most common examples of this are in the fingers and the shoulder joint. Dislocations often cause considerable pain and muscle spasm, cause damage to the joint capsule and surrounding ligaments and may also affect surrounding nerves and muscles. With minor dislocations, it is often difficult for a first aider to tell the difference between a dislocation and a fracture.

Dislocations may also be associated with fractures of nearby bones.

signs

+ Loss of function
+ Swelling at the site
+ Deformity

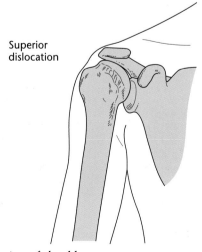

Superior dislocation

Dislocation of shoulder

symptoms

+ Pain and tenderness at the site

treatment

+ Seek medical assistance.
+ Prevent movement occurring at the site of the dislocation to reduce the risk of further tissue damage.
+ Immobilise the injured limb in the position in which you found it, by gently applying a splint and sling. Be sure to immobilise the area above and below the injured joint. Do not attempt to reposition the dislocated joint.
+ Check for signs of circulation below the dislocation. If not present, call for urgent medical assistance.
+ If possible, apply ice packs or cold compresses for between 5 and 15 minutes. Reapply if necessary. This will relieve pain.
+ Treat for shock, as appropriate (see Chapter 7).

NOTE:
- Absence of circulation constitutes a medical emergency. Seek medical aid.
- Do not move the patient until the joint has been immobilised.
- Do not move a patient with an injured hip or dislocated thigh unless it is absolutely necessary.
- Do not test the function of a suspected dislocation.
- Do not attempt to reposition the dislocated joint.
- Do not give the person anything to eat or drink.

subluxation

Subluxations are incomplete dislocations. As with dislocations, subluxations may cause damage to the joint capsule and surrounding ligaments. Treat as for a dislocation.

soft tissue injuries

Soft tissue injuries involve tissues other than bone. With respect to musculoskeletal injuries, they include sprains and strains. If there is doubt about the severity of the injury and whether it involves soft or hard tissue, treat it as a fracture.

strains

A strain is a simple soft tissue injury affecting muscle usually caused by overstretching. Strains will usually heal by themselves, though there may be complications if tendons (which attach muscle to bone) are involved.

signs

+ Swelling
+ Possible discolouration

symptoms

+ Pain on movement

sprains

Sprains are caused when the ligaments that hold bones together are forced beyond their normal range, leading to stretching or tearing. Sprains are more significant injuries than strains and may result in permanent damage if not managed properly.

signs

+ Swelling
+ Loss of power or ability to bear weight
+ Possible discolouration

symptoms

+ Pain (sudden onset)

contusions

A contusion or bruise is a soft tissue injury affecting muscle tissue and blood vessels, which bleed into the muscle. Contusions are usually caused by blunt trauma to the area. Contusions (e.g. a corked thigh) respond well to RICER treatment (see below) and gentle exercise or stretching may be attempted a few hours after the injury.

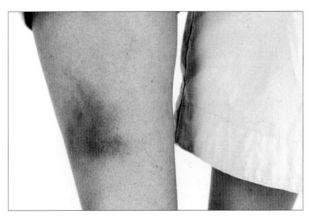

Contusion

signs

+ Swelling
+ Discolouration

symptoms

+ Pain, tenderness at the site of injury

managing soft tissue injuries
RICER

This acronym stands for rest, ice, compression, elevation and referral. This basic approach to soft tissue injuries aims to minimise bleeding, swelling and further tissue damage. Prompt first aid to soft tissue injuries minimises tissue scarring, allowing full recovery and return to daily and sporting activities. Keeping swelling in check early after the injury also enables health care professionals to better diagnose the condition, should medical intervention be necessary.

The principles of RICER

RICER is basic treatment for acute soft tissue injuries and should be used by the first aider in the first 48–72 hours of injury.

Rest

Have the injured person sit or lie down with the injured part supported carefully. Do not allow the patient to move the injured area.

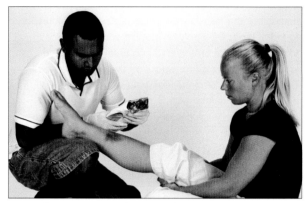

Have the patient rest the injured area

Ice

Use ice or a cold pack to cool the affected area. A polythene bag filled with ice pieces and water is ideal. Wrap this in a damp cloth and place it on the injured site. Apply ice packs (covered by a towel or clothing) or cold compresses for 5–15 minutes; reapply for 5–15 minutes after 5–10 minutes, if necessary, if the area becomes hot or pain recurs. Repeat as required to reduce swelling and pain.

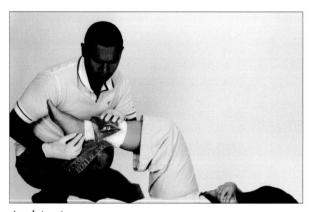

Applying ice

Compression

Apply a compression bandage around the injured area. If using an ice pack, apply the compression bandaging over the ice pack. This will help to support it and reduce movement and swelling at the site of injury. Check circulation is present beyond the bandage to ensure it is not too tight. Also check the colour, warmth, movement and sensation in the area distal to the compression bandage.

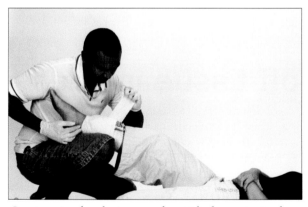

Compression bandaging may be applied over ice packs

Elevation

Raise the injured area above the level of the patient's heart, if possible. This will reduce swelling, bleeding and will help relieve pain.

Referral

Refer the patient to an appropriate health care professional for definitive diagnosis and continuing management. Record the incident, your observations, assessments and treatment given.

In the first 2–3 days after sustaining a soft tissue injury, it is important to do no further HARM.

Do no HARM

Advise the patient to avoid the following for the first 48–72 hours after an injury:

Heat
Any type of heat will increase blood supply to the area and, consequently, bleeding. Avoid hot showers, baths, saunas and do not use hot water bottles or heat rubs.

Alcohol
Consuming alcohol may increase swelling.

Running
Exercising the area too soon may aggravate and worsen the injury. Only contusions should be stretched or gently exercised some hours after the injury.

Massage
Any form of massage will increase swelling and bleeding.

revision

1. List the types of hard tissue injuries:

   a) _____   b) _____   c) _____

2. Complete the following sentences about fractures.

   An .... fracture may be caused by bone piercing the .... and soft tissue when it breaks, or

   from an .... penetrating the skin and fracturing a .... A closed fracture is more ....

   and occurs when the skin remains .... (unbroken).

3. List the signs of a closed fracture:

   a) _____   b) _____   c) _____

   d) _____   e) _____

4. What is the difference between a dislocation and subluxation?

   _____

   _____

5. Complete the following sentences about sprains.

   A strain is a .... soft tissue injury affecting ...., and is usually caused by ....

   Strains will .... heal by themselves, though there may be complications if .... are involved.

6. List the signs and symptoms of a sprain:

   a) _____   b) _____

   c) _____   d) _____

7. What does the acronym RICER stand for?

   R: _____

   I: _____

   C: _____

   E: _____

   R: _____

8. What is meant by do no HARM for 3 days after the injury?

   H: _____

   A: _____

   R: _____

   M: _____

Answers appear in Appendix 8.

moving injured casualties

learning outcomes

Perform the correct method of moving injured casualties.

+ Detail the factors to be considered prior to moving a casualty.
+ Demonstrate the correct method for lifting and carrying a casualty.
+ Detail the methods of moving a casualty.

how you may be assessed

underpinning knowledge

A number of oral or written questions may be asked relating to considerations prior to moving a casualty, correct lifts and carries and the various methods of moving a casualty. Examples have been included at the end of the chapter.

practical demonstration

You may be asked to show what factors you would consider prior to moving a casualty. You may be required to demonstrate the correct method of lifting or carrying a casualty.

scenario

You may be required to carry or move one or more patients who have different injuries and first aid needs.

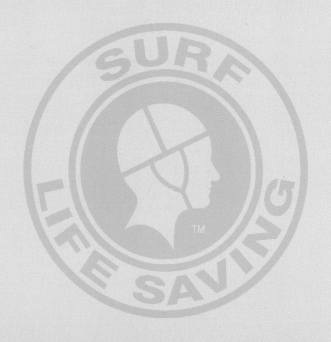

In the absence of medical help, moving a casualty should only be attempted when the patient is in immediate or imminent danger, as any movement may worsen their injury. Rescuing a patient from water is one example, where the patient needs to be moved on to land for safety, treatment or resuscitation. In the event that the patient must be moved, it is important to select an appropriate method of movement for the safety of the patient and the first aider.

considerations prior to moving a casualty

+ Danger
+ Location
+ Route of movement
+ Equipment
+ Personnel
+ Urgency
+ Safe methods of lifting and carrying

lifting and carrying

+ Face in the direction you intend to lift and move.
+ Bend the knees and crouch down, keeping your back straight.
+ Balancing with a wide base of support (knees about shoulder width apart), take secure hold of the object to be lifted.
+ Keep the load close to the body, if possible.
+ One member should co-ordinate the lift and instruct other members on when and how to lift.
+ Brace your stomach muscles and, with your back in an upright position, lift the object using your legs.

NOTE:
Do not bend forward with straight legs to lift. This places excessive load on your lower back.

methods of moving a casualty

Patients should be moved with the greatest of care. For patients with suspected spinal injury, see Chapter 21 for specific methods of carrying.

stretcher

Seriously injured patients should be moved by stretcher to prevent further injury and patients in shock should be moved very carefully to avoid cardiac problems.

Other types of immobilisation (e.g. cervical collar, splints, etc) should be applied before moving patients by stretcher.

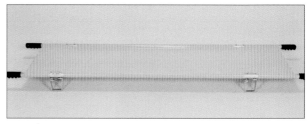
Stretcher

scoop

An advantage of scoop stretchers is that they are assembled underneath the patient without having to move the patient.

+ Lay the stretcher beside the patient and adjust for the patient's height.
+ Detach both ends of the stretcher.
+ Slide both halves of the stretcher underneath the patient and re-attach both ends. The head end should be re-attached first, so the person at this end can

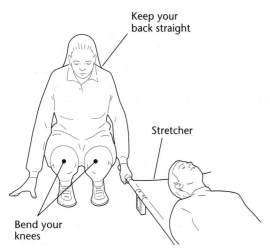
How to lift

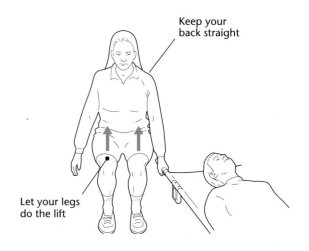

stabilise the head while the foot end is re-attached by another first aider or a bystander.

✚ The patient is ready to be moved, using appropriate lifting techniques, to ensure no injury to the rescuers.

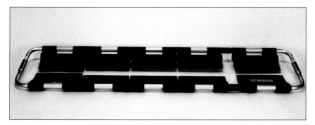

Aussie scoop

spinal board

Spinal boards are hard and rigid, rectangular in shape with handles along the sides. Mostly designed to be buoyant for aquatic emergencies, spinal boards are designed to stabilise the spine and head in a neutral position (see Chapter 21).

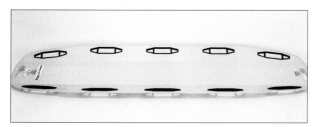

Ambulance stretcher

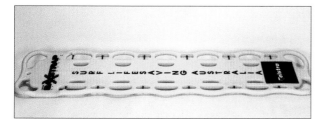

Baxstrap spine board

blankets

Blankets can be used as an emergency stretcher. There are some special considerations to adhere to when lifting and carrying using a blanket as a stretcher.

✚ The blanket needs to be of adequate strength and length to extend beyond the patient's head and feet. Test the blanket's strength by placing a non-injured party on the blanket and conducting a trial lift.

✚ Roll up the blanket along its length (i.e. from side to side, not top to bottom) until half the blanket is flat on the ground.

✚ While the patient is being rolled on their side, the rolled edged is then placed along the patient's side. As close to the patient's body as possible.

✚ Carefully, roll the patient onto the blanket.

✚ Roll blankets edges in towards patient's body.

✚ Using the rolled edges for grip, carefully lift and move the patient as a team.

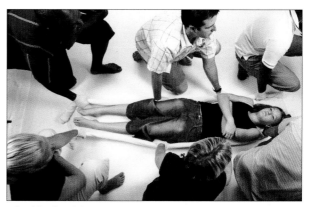

The blanket lift

non-stretcher
one-person human crutch

This assisted walk is appropriate for conscious patients who are capable of standing, as long as they do not have arm or upper body injuries.

✚ The first aider stands beside the patient. The patient places one arm over the first aider's shoulder, which the first aider holds to secure the patient.

✚ The first aider supports the patient around the waist with the arm closest to the patient.

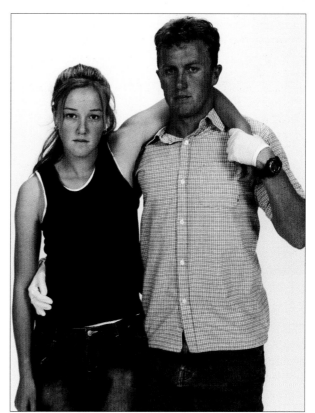

One-person human crutch

two-person human crutch

This assisted walk is particularly suitable for patients who cannot support their weight.

✚ Two first aiders stand either side of the patient. The patient places an arm over each of the first aiders' shoulders. The first aiders hold the patient's hands to secure the position.

✚ Each first aider places their free arm around the patient's waist for support.

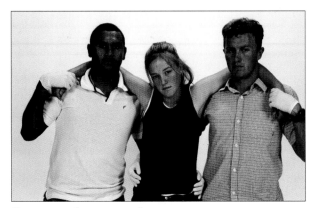

Two-person human crutch

two-handed seat

This method is suitable for unconscious or disoriented patients or those with arm or upper body injuries. It requires two people to support the patient.

✚ Two first aiders stand facing each other behind the patient.
✚ Arms are locked at the wrist under the patient's knees and behind the patient's back.
✚ The first aiders should stand at the same time, taking care to keep their backs straight. They should start walking with the outside leg.

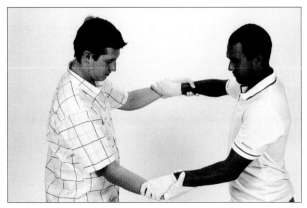

Two-handed seat

four-handed seat

This method is suitable for conscious patients who are capable of holding on to one or both first aiders, but unable to bear weight or stand upright. It requires two people to support the patient.

✚ Two first aiders stand facing each other behind the patient. Each holds their own left wrist with their right hand and grasps the other first aider's right wrist with their left hand creating the 'seat'.
✚ Squatting down, bring the four-handed seat under the patient.
✚ Ask the patient to place their arms around the first aiders' necks.
✚ The first aiders should stand at the same time, taking care to keep their backs straight. They should start walking with the outside leg.

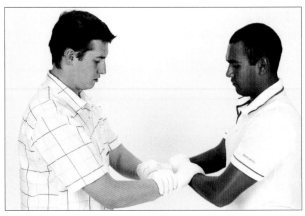

Four-handed seat

emergency drags

In emergency situations, a patient may be moved via one of the following methods:

✚ arm drag
✚ leg drag
✚ clothing drag.

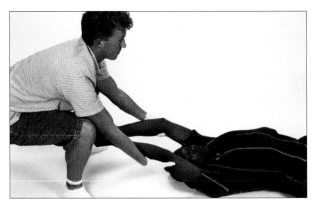

Arm drag

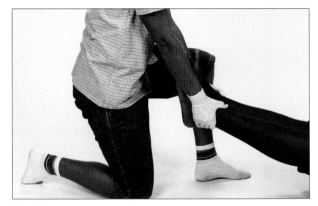

Leg drag

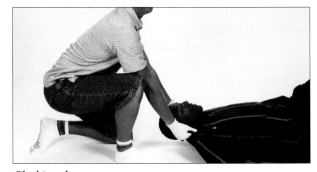

Clothing drag

revision

1. Complete the following sentence about moving injured casualties.

    In the absence of .... help, moving a casualty should only be .... when the patient is in

    immediate or .... danger, as any .... may .... their injury.

2. List five factors that you should consider before moving a casualty:

    a) _____ b) _____ c) _____

    d) _____ e) _____

3. List three stretcher methods of moving a casualty:

    a) _____ b) _____ c) _____

4. List five non-stretcher methods of moving a casualty:

    a) _____

    b) _____

    c) _____

    d) _____

    e) _____

5. Indicate the correct sequence of events for a four-handed seat carry:

    ___ Ask the patient to place their arms around the first aiders' necks.

    ___ The first aiders should stand at the same time and start walking with the outside leg.

    ___ Two first aiders stand facing each other behind the patient.

    ___ Each first aider holds their own left wrist with their right hand and grasps the other first aider's right wrist with their left hand creating the 'seat'.

    ___ Squatting down, bring the four-handed seat under the patient.

Answers appear in Appendix 8.

chapter eighteen | moving injured casualties

drug and substance abuse

learning outcomes

Perform first aid for drug and substance abuse.

+ Describe some of the classification systems used for drugs.
+ Detail the effects drugs may have on the human body.
+ Detail the availability of drugs in the community.

how you may be assessed

underpinning knowledge

A number of oral or written questions may be asked relating to drug classification, effects of drugs on the human body and the availability of drugs in the community. Examples have been included at the end of the chapter.

practical demonstration

You may be required to demonstrate how you would identify a patient suspected of drug and/or substance abuse.

scenario

You may be required to demonstrate how you would identify one or more patients suspected of drug and/or substance abuse.

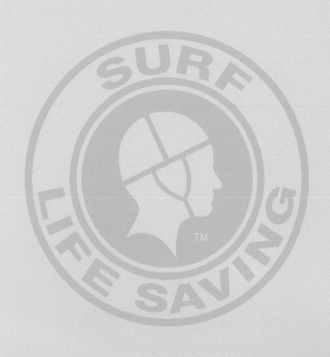

Drug and substance abuse includes the abuse and overdose of illicit, prescription and non-prescription medication and other substances (e.g. petrol and glue) in a manner not intended by the manufacturer or in doses above those recommended. The reasons for drug or substance use and abuse are many and varied, and drugs and substances may be used recreationally, chronically or to inflict intentional self-harm or attempt suicide. All drugs, whether legal or illegal, have some sort of side effects and the legal status in no way reflects the amount of harm they may cause. Side effects depend on the type of drug, the amount taken, the metabolism of the person using the drug and whether the drug is used in conjunction with any other drugs.

what is a drug?

A drug is any substance that, when it enters the body, changes the way a person's mind and/or body functions.

classification of drugs

Drugs can be classified either by the effect they have on the body or their availability to the population (legal status).

effect

There are many different classes of drugs with varying effects on the body. However, the first aider is most likely to come in contact with people using stimulants, hallucinogens and depressants.

stimulants

These are drugs that have the ability to increase activity in the central nervous system. They often make a person feel more alert and confident, but may also cause over-stimulation.

Stimulant drugs can have the following effects on the human body:

+ increase alertness and mask the signs of fatigue
+ produce feelings of euphoria and increased well-being
+ cause anxiety and bizarre behaviour
+ increase heart rate
+ increase blood pressure (constriction of blood vessels)
+ increase respiratory rate
+ dilate pupils
+ suppress appetite
+ insomnia.

Some common stimulant drugs include:

+ caffeine: found in coffee, tea, cola soft drinks, caffeine-containing 'energy' drinks, fatigue-reduction medications
+ nicotine: found in tobacco products
+ amphetamines: e.g. speed, ecstasy, benzedrine, dexedrine
+ cocaine: made from the erythroxylon coca bush. Also known as coke
+ crack: a crystallised freebase form of cocaine. Named after the sound produced when being smoked.

depressants

These are drugs that have the ability to slow down activity in the central nervous system. They have a calming and relaxing effect on the body in low doses and adversely affect co-ordination and concentration. In large doses depressants can cause generalised inco-ordination, slurred speech, nausea and vomiting and may cause unconsciousness by reducing breathing and heart rate. Different classes of depressants should not be taken together as their effects are exacerbated, increasing the risk of overdose.

Depressant drugs can have the following effects on the human body:

+ analgesia (pain reduction)
+ anaesthesia (loss of sensation)
+ decrease heart rate

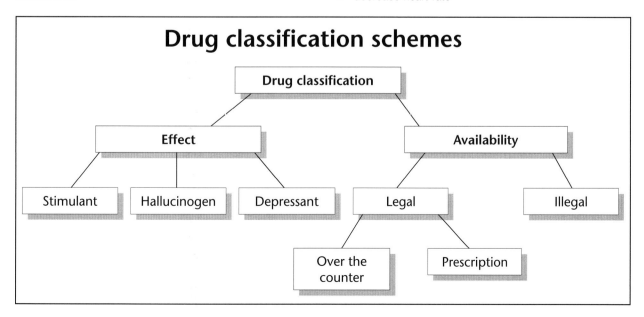

- decrease respiratory rate
- relief from anxiety
- sedation
- produce feelings of euphoria and increased well-being.

Some common depressant drugs include:

- alcohol
- narcotic analgesics: found in opium products, e.g. heroin, morphine, codeine
- general anaesthetics: surgical anaesthetics and inhaled anaesthetics (e.g. nitrous oxide [Entonox], methoxyflurane [Penthrox]; see Chapter 25)
- sedative hypnotics: e.g. barbiturates, benzodiazepines (tranquillisers)
- cannabis: found in the *Cannabis sativa* plant. Also called hashish or marijuana.

hallucinogens

Hallucinogenic (or psychedelic) drugs alter a person's perception of reality. They affect all the senses and can also markedly alter mood and thought.

Hallucinogenic drugs can have a variety of effects on the body and are subjective to the drug user. Reactions can range from feelings of dread and terror (a bad trip) to extreme euphoria.

Some common hallucinogenic drugs include:

- marijuana/hashish (in high doses): found in the *Cannabis sativa* plant. It also has depressant effects in small amounts
- LSD (lysergic acid diethylamide, 'trips'): made in home-made laboratories
- mescaline: found in products made from the Mexican peyote cactus
- psylocybin (magic mushrooms): found in products made from the psylocybe and conocybe mushroom
- PCP (phenylcyclidine): angel dust
- ecstasy.

availability
illegal

Some drugs are banned from use by the general public as they can have dangerous consequences if not used for their intended purpose, while others are classified as illegal or illicit because they are deemed to have little or no medicinal value. Illicit drugs have no quality controls dictating their manufacture, price or distribution. As such, the strength, purity and availability of a particular drug are unpredictable and can result in considerable harm to the user. Unintentional overdose may result from unpredictable purity of drugs such as heroin, and additives to any illicit drugs can be poisonous, and may result in injury and even death.

legal

The majority of the population can purchase legal drugs. Certain laws may restrict their sale to people of a certain age (e.g. alcohol, tobacco). They can also be available 'over the counter' or via a medical practitioner's prescription.

prescription

These drugs can only be purchased with a doctor's prescription and they are used to treat a specific health problem or condition. They should only be used for their intended purpose (e.g. antibiotics for infection, tranquillisers for anxiety or panic disorders and psychosis) and at the dosage indicated.

over the counter

These drugs can be purchased from shops or pharmacies without a prescription. They are used to promote health (e.g. vitamin and mineral supplements, herbals, homeopathics, etc) or treat minor pain and illness. They can still cause harmful effects if not used for their intended purpose (e.g. mild analgesics such as aspirin and paracetamol can be dangerous in overdose).

For information on identifying and treating drug and substance abuse, please refer to Chapter 14

revision

1. Complete the following sentence about drug and substance abuse.

    Drug and substance abuse includes the abuse and overdose of .... prescription and ....

    medication and other .... in a manner not intended by the .... or in doses above those

    ....

2. List five effects of stimulant drugs:

    a) _____

    b) _____

    c) _____

    d) _____

    e) _____

3. List five common stimulant drugs:

    a) _____   b) _____   c) _____

    d) _____   e) _____

4. List five effects of depressant drugs:

    a) _____

    b) _____

    c) _____

    d) _____

    e) _____

5. List five common depressant drugs:

    a) _____   b) _____   c) _____

    d) _____   e) _____

6. List five hallucinogenic drugs:

    a) _____

    b) _____

    c) _____

    d) _____

    e) _____

Answers appear in Appendix 8.

drug and substance abuse

emergency childbirth

learning outcomes

Perform first aid for emergency childbirth.

+ Detail how to assist with the delivery of a baby.
+ Detail how to protect against infection during emergency childbirth.
+ Describe the three phases of labour.
+ Describe how to assist when there are cord complications during emergency childbirth.
+ Detail the care of the newborn infant after emergency childbirth.
+ Detail the complications that can occur during pregnancy that may require first aid and emergency care.

how you may be assessed

underpinning knowledge

A number of oral or written questions may be asked relating to delivery of a baby, possible infection during delivery, phases of labour, cord complications, care of newborn infants and complications that may be experienced during pregnancy. Examples have been included at the end of the chapter.

practical demonstration

You may be asked to demonstrate what you would do to assist with the delivery of a baby. You may be asked to show how you would assist when there are cord complications during childbirth. You may be asked to show what care must be taken of a newborn infant after emergency childbirth. You may be asked to show what first aid and emergency care may be required in the event of a complication during pregnancy.

scenario

You may be required to simulate assisting a woman in labour without immediate medical assistance, when childbirth is imminent.

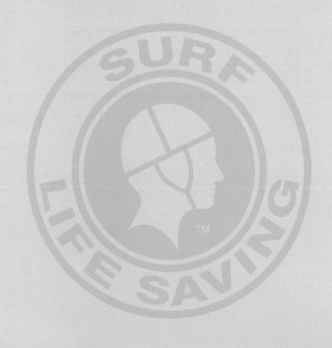

A first aider will rarely be called upon to assist with childbirth. It should not be feared as, generally, emergency childbirth is due to a very rapid labour, especially if this is not the mother's first labour, indicating that everything is progressing well. The exception to this is, of course, premature labour.

Knowing the stages of labour and what to expect will provide the first aider with enough confidence to support and reassure the mother-to-be, assist her deliver her baby and keep both mother and baby safe until medical help arrives.

how to assist

There are several steps that can be taken to assist with the delivery of a baby if childbirth is imminent before medical assistance can arrive. In all circumstances, an attempt should be made to contact or seek professional medical assistance as a matter of urgency.

Steps in assisting with an emergency childbirth include:

+ calling for an ambulance
+ protecting the mother and child from infection
+ assisting with the birth of the baby
+ caring for the newborn infant
+ delivery of the placenta.

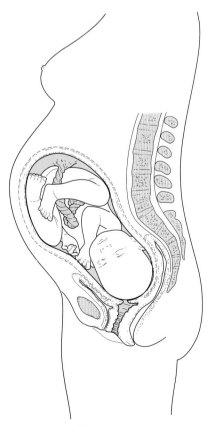

The usual position of the baby at full-term

infection control

The process of childbirth can leave mother and infant exposed to infection. During childbirth, involuntary bowel movements are common as the baby descends through the vagina, thereby expelling any faecal matter in the rectum. As the anus is very close to the vaginal opening, through which the baby is delivered, it is very important that you take all possible precautions in protecting the mother and baby against infection from both your actions and the surrounding environment.

Where possible, sterile medical gloves should be worn during the entire process. If gloves are unavailable, a thorough hand scrub with soap and warm water will be required. Wearing a mask is also strongly advised.

Any precautions you can take to make the surrounding environment as clean as possible will also assist in preventing infection. While the use of clean sheets, sheets of plastic and towels will be of benefit during the childbirth process, this is often impractical in an emergency situation. Clean (sterile) string that can be used for umbilical ties and a pair of sharp (sterile) scissors will be useful, but often unobtainable. If possible, they may need to be boiled in order to sterilise them.

stage 1 labour

There are three phases to the first stage of labour:

+ early phase (including the onset of labour)
+ active phase
+ transition.

The onset of labour is variable. It is usually a longer process for first-time mothers allowing time for medical care to arrive. However, this is not always the case, especially for subsequent pregnancies and delivery may take place before medical help is available. Labour may start with more obscure symptoms like period cramps or back pain or the minor contractions felt may be difficult to distinguish from the non-painful Braxton-Hicks contractions. As this phase progresses, the contractions become stronger and more painful.

During stage one there is mucous discharge from the vagina that becomes more blood-stained as the contractions become more intense and small vessels in the cervix rupture as it thins and opens. There may also be a 'show' if this did not present before labour. This is the blood-stained mucous plug that plugged the cervix during pregnancy. The waters (amniotic fluid surrounding the baby inside the amniotic sac) may break during this phase as either a trickle or a gush. There is no clear time frame on the show or waters breaking — the gap between the two events may be many days or at the last minute before the baby is delivered.

During the active phase the contractions are very painful as they work towards thinning (effacing) and opening (dilating) the cervix. A good sign that labour is active is that the mother probably can't talk through the contractions.

The final phase of stage one labour is transition, which is the most intense phase of labour. Contractions will be very intense and long (up to around 60 seconds) as the cervix dilates to 10 cm. The mother may be very tired, emotional, anxious and may lose focus and feel overwhelmed and unable to cope during this phase. Reassurance is especially important for the mother, as is the knowledge that delivery of the baby is getting close.

At this stage of the process, it is important to stay calm, constantly reassure the mother and clean the area under and around her using clean linen — towels or sheets where possible. You then need to position yourself and the mother for delivery. The mother will know which position is most comfortable for her. If possible, it is best to keep the mother's buttocks elevated somehow (e.g. over the edge of a bed or table) so you can deliver the baby's shoulders and so a basin or similar can be placed beneath her to collect any amniotic fluid and blood during the birth. Remove any unnecessary clothing to make the mother comfortable and to permit delivery of the baby. The first aider will need to be in a position to observe the birth canal and monitor the mother's progress.

sation that she will open her bowels, which most women do, as the baby's head begins its descent through the vagina. Many women experience renewed energy during this stage and the contractions may be further apart now, allowing time to rest between them. At this point ask the mother *not* to push, but rather pant to help delay the birth and allow more time for medical help to arrive.

If the baby begins to appear, the top of the head should appear first. This process is known as 'crowning'. If the 'waters' have not broken yet, nick the amniotic sac covering the baby's head with something sharp and sterile, if possible, taking care to avoid the face. If the bottom appears first, keep trying to delay the birth by advising the mother to keep panting and not to push. See 'complications requiring first aid'.

As 'crowning' occurs, urge the woman not to push and just pant, while assisting delivery of the head by applying gentle counter-pressure to try to avoid an 'explosive' birth, which can damage the woman's perineum (area between the anus and the vagina). When the head is delivered, you will need to feel under the baby's chin for the umbilical cord, which may be wrapped around the baby's neck, but tell the mother before you do so, as this will probably be painful for her.

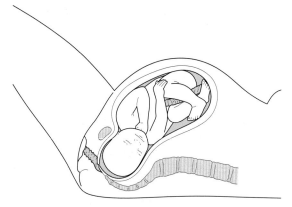

Stage 1 labour

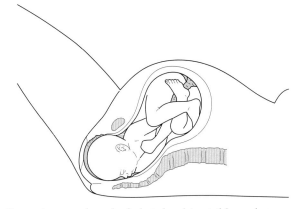

Crowning — when the baby's head is visible at the vaginal opening

stage 2 labour — birth of the baby

By now the cervix is fully effaced and fully dilated and by the end of this stage, the baby will be born. The mother-to-be may feel the urge to push now and have the sen-

If the umbilical cord is around the neck, ask the mother to keep panting while you slide one or two fingers under the cord and gently lever it over the baby's head. There is usually enough slack in the umbilical cord to permit this. If this is not possible, assist with the delivery of the rest of the baby and remove it as soon as possible

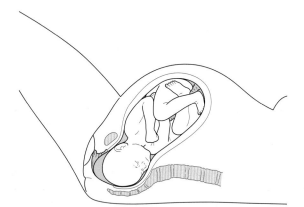

Stage 2 labour

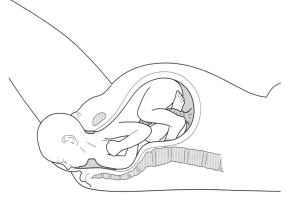

Delivery of the head

after delivering the body. After the head is delivered it usually spontaneously rotates to face sideways. Place your hands either side of the head and very gently guide the head and neck downwards (but do *not* pull the head). This movement will assist the top shoulder to emerge. You may need to ask the mother to push to assist this process.

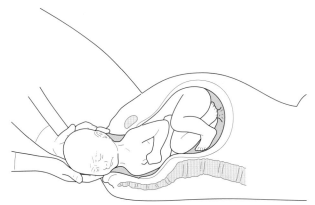

Gently guide the head down (without pulling) to assist delivery of the shoulders

NOTE:
- Do not try and inhibit delivery of the baby other than asking the mother to pant rather than push.
- Do not pull on the baby's head to speed delivery of the body.
- Do not pull on the umbilical cord.

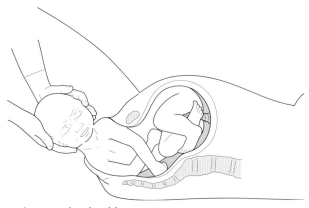

Delivering the shoulders

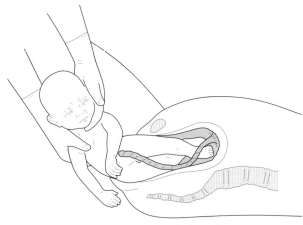

By the end of stage 2 labour, the baby is born

Usually, one more gentle push from the mother will deliver the other shoulder and the rest of the body with it.

cord complications

In some instances where the cord is very firmly around the baby's neck and cannot be levered over the head, the infant may be at risk of cerebral hypoxia, so the cord needs to be clamped and tied as a matter of urgency. A sign of foetal distress is falling heart rate, though the first aider cannot monitor foetal reactions, so judgement is critical.

Tie the cord off firmly, with sterile string or similar, in two places above and two places below the area to be cut. Check the ties are firmly tied as, if they are not done correctly, life-threatening bleeding can occur. Ensure the cord is cut between the two ties above and the two ties below.

The baby needs to be delivered as quickly as possible, as it is not receiving oxygenated blood from the mother and an airway needs to be established immediately. If the baby does not begin breathing spontaneously, start EAR and CPR, as appropriate (see Chapters 4, 5).

NOTE:
If any complication occurs, cutting the cord is always best left to a medical professional.

care of the newborn infant

Note the time the baby is born. Newborns lose body temperature rapidly and must be protected from hypothermia. Firstly, dry and wrap the baby in a clean warm blanket (covering the head, but not the face) and give to the mother to hold. Congratulate the mother on a job well done! If possible, clean the baby's mouth and nose with a soft cotton swab. Do not interfere with the umbilical cord. Encourage the mother to try and breastfeed the baby (if she intends to) to assist uterine contractions and delivery of the placenta.

Often, a newborn is not breathing immediately after childbirth and gentle stimulation of the skin and body may assist breathing to start: if not, gently tap the bottom of the baby's feet. After one minute, if the baby appears not to be breathing, clear the airway and begin EAR with gentle puffs of air and check if the umbilical cord is beating. If it is, then it is delivering blood to the baby and CPR is unnecessary. If the cord is not beating and the baby has no pulse, start CPR.

After 2–3 minutes, the umbilical cord will stop pulsating as the baby's heart takes over. At this point the baby is no longer dependent on the mother's circulatory system. If you are confident in what you are doing and have sterile ties then apply them around the umbilical cord at approximately 12 cm, 15 cm, 20 cm and 23 cm from the baby's navel. The ties need to be tied firmly enough to stop any blood flow from the baby. There is no need to cut the cord, especially if there are no sterile scissors or scalpel to do so — no harm can be done leaving it secured to the baby until medical help arrives. If the cord is cut, it needs to be done between the 15 cm and 20 cm tie, i.e. leaving two ties on the baby side of the umbilical cord.

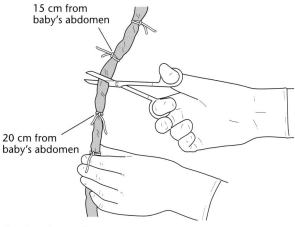

15 cm from baby's abdomen

20 cm from baby's abdomen

Cutting the cord

If possible, note the condition of the baby at 1 and 5 minutes after delivery to approximate an APGAR score (see Appendix 6).

stage 3 labour – delivery of the placenta

After the baby has been delivered, the placenta will be expelled any time from 10 minutes to one hour later.

Position yourself where you can observe the birth canal, mother and infant. Once the placenta has been delivered, try and store the placenta in a plastic bag or container and place it in a refrigerator, if possible. This will allow the placenta to be examined by medical staff at a later time to ensure it is intact (i.e. that the whole placenta has been delivered and that none remains in the uterus to cause bleeding or infection).

Once the placenta has been expelled and the umbilical cord has stopped pulsating, the baby is breathing and circulating oxygen-rich blood on its own, without assistance from the mother. It is important to keep reassuring the mother until medical assistance arrives. Allow the mother to have a drink to replace the fluids she will have lost during the delivery. Provide the mother

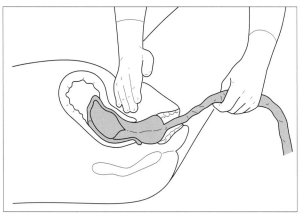

Delivery of the placenta

with sanitary napkins, if available, or some absorbent dressing, as vaginal bleeding will continue due to separation of the placenta from the wall of the uterus.

Check for excessive vaginal bleeding (haemorrhage). Average blood loss during a normal vaginal delivery is 300–500 mL. If blood loss is excessive, treat the mother for shock. Retain all collected fluids and material soiled with blood for examination by medical staff.

Keep the mother and baby warm until medical help arrives. Both the mother and baby will need to be checked out at hospital to ensure there are no complications from the delivery.

> **+ NOTE:**
> Only cut the umbilical cord if:
> • the baby requires resuscitation
> • the mother needs urgent care
> • the placenta is not delivered within 60 minutes of the baby being delivered.

complications requiring first aid

There are several complications that can occur during a pregnancy and childbirth that may require assistance from a first aider. If either of the following occur, you will need to seek additional medical assistance immediately.

breech birth

If, during the crowning process, a baby's foot or buttocks appear rather than the top of the head, you will be dealing with a 'breech birth'. It is important to calm the mother and try and delay the birth by telling her to pant rather than push.

In all cases, monitor the mother for heavy bleeding from the birth canal that may cause shock: if it occurs, treat accordingly (see Chapter 7). If the mother loses consciousness, place her on her left side and follow the directions for resuscitation during pregnancy (see Chapter 5).

miscarriage in early pregnancy

If a woman is experiencing a miscarriage, there will be heavy vaginal bleeding and severe cramps in the lower abdomen. Seek medical assistance as a priority, followed by allowing the casualty to rest in a comfortable position. You may need to place a pillow under their knees to ease abdominal pain. Offer constant reassurance.

You will also need to monitor the casualty's vital signs very carefully, noting changes in breathing and pulse rate. If breathing rate and pulse rate begin to deteriorate, you may need to treat the patient for shock (see Chapter 7). Provide plenty of reassurance to the patient until help arrives and avoid giving the patient anything to eat or drink as they may require surgery once they get to hospital.

revision

1. What are the steps a first aider can take to assist with emergency childbirth?

    a) _____

    b) _____

    c) _____

    d) _____

    e) _____

2. What are the three phases of stage one labour?

    a) _____   b) _____   c) _____

3. Describe the changes to the cervix that occur during stage one labour.

    _____

    _____

    _____

4. Which of the following statements about care of the newborn infant is *not* entirely true?
    a) You should protect the baby against hypothermia.
    b) If the newborn is not breathing on delivery, firmly smack the baby' bottom to stimulate breathing.
    c) While the umbilical cord is still pulsating, the baby is receiving blood from the mother.
    d) In an uncomplicated delivery there is no urgency to cut the cord.

5. Define breech birth.

    _____

    _____

Answers appear in Appendix 8.

spinal injuries and management

learning outcomes

Perform first aid for the management of spinal injuries.

+ Describe the possible causes of spinal injuries.
+ Detail the signs and symptoms of a patient with suspected spinal injuries.
+ Demonstrate how to move a patient with suspected spinal injuries.
+ Detail the principles of immobilisation for spinal injuries.
+ Detail the management of head and spinal injuries.
+ Demonstrate the management of head and spinal injuries.
+ Detail the precautions necessary for the transportation of patients with suspected spinal injuries.

how you may be assessed

underpinning knowledge

A number of oral or written questions may be asked relating to the causes, signs and symptoms of spinal injuries, moving patients with suspected spinal injuries, immobilisation, identification and treatment of head injuries and the transportation of patients with suspected spinal injuries. Examples have been included at the end of the chapter.

practical demonstration

You may be asked to demonstrate how you would move a casualty with a suspected spinal injury. You may be asked to demonstrate how you would manage a patient with head and spinal injuries. You may be asked to demonstrate the precautions necessary for the transportation of patients with suspected spinal injuries.

scenario

You may be required to treat one or more patients who have suspected head and/or spinal injuries.

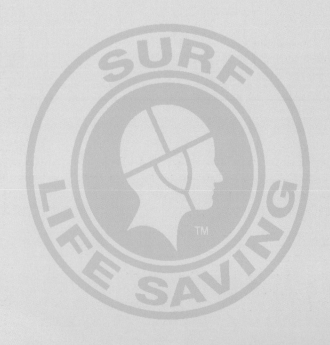

spinal injuries

Spinal injuries can result from a number of activities, with motor vehicle accidents and diving emergencies accounting for most injuries. With proper management, if the spinal cord has not been severed or damaged on initial impact, it can be protected against further trauma. Unless an accident has been witnessed, or if a neck and/or back injury is highly improbable, you should always treat motionless and unconscious patients for a spinal injury. A first aider should always inspect the scene to identify any possible causes that may have contributed to the accident. These may be:

+ motor vehicle accident
+ industrial accident (workplace)
+ diving accident
+ sporting accident (e.g. rugby scrum, falling from a horse)
+ a fall from a height
+ a significant blow to the head (from a blunt force)
+ severe penetrating wounds (i.e. gunshot, stabbing, etc).

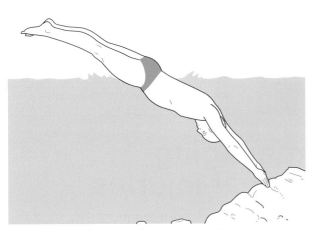
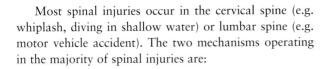

Be aware of submerged obstacles when diving into shallow water

Most spinal injuries occur in the cervical spine (e.g. whiplash, diving in shallow water) or lumbar spine (e.g. motor vehicle accident). The two mechanisms operating in the majority of spinal injuries are:

+ vertical compression
+ forward bending (flexion) with rotation.

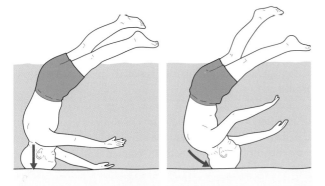

Vertical compression and forward flexion of the neck

As a result of this type of injury (a minority of injuries are due to extension), ligaments may be broken and vertebrae fractured or dislocated. It is very difficult to determine the severity of a spinal injury without an X-ray.

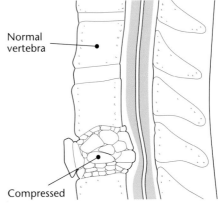

A wedge compression fracture resulting in pressure on the spinal cord

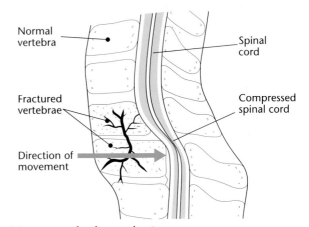

Movement of a damaged spine

signs

+ Breathing difficulties
+ Profuse bleeding from the head, or abrasions, or bruising to the forehead
+ Dilated pupils
+ Fluid leaking from the ears
+ Abnormal blood pressure
+ Shock
+ Loss of consciousness

symptoms

+ Back or neck pain
+ Tingling or lack of feeling in lower or upper limbs
+ Increased muscle tone (muscles become more rigid)
+ Dizziness
+ Headache

NOTE:
Patients with head trauma may also have sustained spinal injuries.

moving casualties with suspected spinal injuries

When a casualty is found lying in an awkward or unusual position on the ground (usually from a fall from a height), they should not be moved unless under the supervision of an experienced rescue and/or health care worker with specific equipment.

This may not be possible if the person is at further risk of danger (e.g. surf, fire, etc). In this case, the basic principles of managing spinal injuries need to be followed and adapted. When moving such patients, the priorities are:

✚ airway and circulation
✚ minimising movement of the head and cervical spine
✚ minimising movement of the thoracic and lumbar spine, sacrum and coccyx.

The patient should be moved the shortest distance to a safe position. At all stages of the move, the body should be manipulated in a way that the head, neck and spine are immobilised as one body part. The patient's arms and legs should be moved first if any body part has to be moved. Arms should be placed above the head or alongside the body in an attempt to roll the patient like a 'log'. Ideally, the patient should be fitted with a cervical collar or placed on a spinal board.

principles of immobilisation

Due to the unknown severity of any spinal injury, all suspected cases should be treated as life-threatening. Providing appropriate emergency care in this situation can help prevent further injury to the spinal cord and, in cases of higher cervical damage (where respiratory muscles are paralysed), may save lives. When assisting patients with a suspected spinal injury, one of the most important factors, other than the care of the airway, is immobilisation.

Immobilisation should be attempted on a suspected spinal injury as soon as possible. The main aims of spinal immobilisation are to ensure that the head and spine remain in a neutral position, and to avoid or minimise movement, which may cause further harm.

improvised spinal management

Ideally, the most effective form of immobilisation is with the use of a cervical collar and specific spinal board, but these may not always be available. Some of the following methods can assist in the temporary immobilisation of a patient until further medical aid arrives:

✚ hands gently holding the head in the neutral position
✚ packing of sand, dirt, towels, newspaper around the patient to prevent movement.

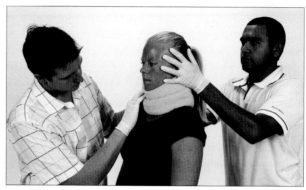

An improvised cervical collar using a towel

NOTE:
- Improvised immobilisation techniques should only be attempted by a first aider who is confident in their ability, because movement may cause further injury.
- If a first aider is not confident with the situation, the patient should be left in the position found and monitored and comforted however possible.

managing spinal injuries

Managing head and spinal injuries involves supporting the respiratory, circulatory, skeletal and nervous systems. When treating and managing a patient with a suspected spinal injury, the following key principles should be considered:

✚ danger
✚ level of consciousness
✚ airway management
✚ immobilisation
✚ treatment
✚ stabilisation.

the cervical collar

A cervical collar is designed to minimise movement and, therefore, the risk of further injury to the spinal cord. The collar — a foam and plastic device — is designed to assist in maintaining the cervical spine in a neutral position.

Cervical collars come in a range of sizes to suit different body shapes and sizes. One-size-fits-all collars should only be used if they are adjustable. Collars should only be fitted and applied by trained and experienced personnel.

fitting the collar

✚ Ensure the head is maintained in the neutral position, unless, due to the nature of the injury, this is not possible.

✚ Determine the 'key dimension', which determines the size of the cervical collar to use for the patient.

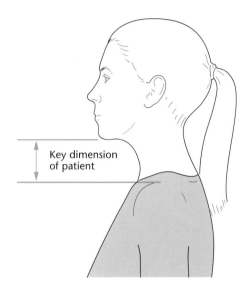

Measuring the key dimension

✚ Select or adjust the cervical collar to ensure that the key dimension measurement taken from the neck can be accommodated.

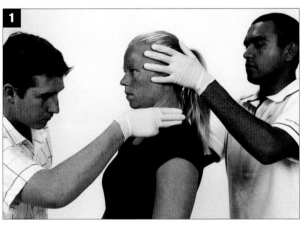

Adjusting a cervical collar to the key dimension

✚ Gently slide the collar up the patient's chest and neck, being careful to ensure that there is no pressure placed on the trachea. If the back of the patient's neck is obstructed by something, such as a car seat or the ground, etc, the collar should be slid under the back of the neck first with the velcro strip folded back.

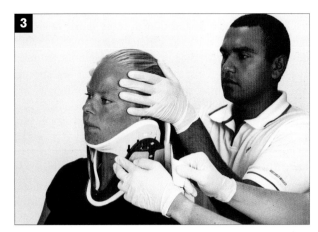

Fitting a cervical collar

✚ Pass the strap underneath the patient's neck and secure in position with velcro fasteners.

✚ Ensure that the collar has been fitted in the neutral position and is a snug fit around the neck, preventing movement.

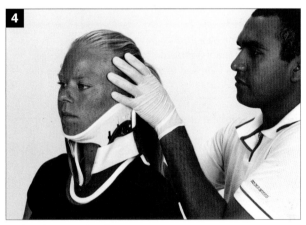

A fitted cervical collar

✚ Monitor the patient constantly and continue with spinal management.

NOTE:
Remember that a cervical collar is only an aid in spinal management and should not be used as the only form of treatment.

spinal boards

Along with cervical collars, spinal boards and head blocks are the best means of spinal immobilisation. Spinal boards are hard, rigid and rectangular in shape with handles along the sides. Spinal boards are designed to stabilise the spine and head in a neutral position. Most spinal boards have body straps attached for immobilising the patient and the facility to attach some form of head immobilisation. Spinal boards and head blocks, which are strongly recommended for virtually all cases of suspected spinal injury, should only be used by trained personnel.

The design and application of most spinal boards is fairly generic. In contrast, different head blocks, while designed around the same principles, have different operating procedures. This chapter briefly describes specific head blocks and their application. For further details and instructions, consult the relevant product manuals.

head immobilisation blocks

Laerdal SpeedBlocks

The Laerdal SpeedBlocks system allows variable adjustment to suit each individual's head and neck shape (from 2 years and up). This system consists of a backing board and two securing plates made of plastic and velcro, with disposable head pads and straps. SpeedBlocks use a push-and-lock system for adjustment and are secured with velcro straps across the chin and forehead.

+ With the patient lying on the spinal board with their head in the neutral position over the disposable foam pad, place the blocks either side of their head.
+ SpeedBlocks are attached by squeezing in the grey tabs and placing the head blocks on top of the sliding rails.
+ Once in the sliding rails, push the SpeedBlocks together slowly and safely to secure the head.
+ Secure the forehead and chin straps over the patient's face.

Once applied, the SpeedBlocks should minimise movement of the head and cervical spine. SpeedBlocks do not need to be removed for imaging (X-ray, CT or MRI).

spinal stretcher immobilisation

In patients with a suspected spinal injury, all due care should be taken to limit the movement of the spine when managing the airway. However, management of the airway takes precedence over management of the spinal injury.

for conscious or prone patients on land

The following steps apply to spinal stretcher immobilisation in conscious or prone patients managed on land.

+ If possible, maintain and support the head in the neutral position by placing your hands either side of the patient's head.
+ A cervical collar should be fitted and applied by trained personnel only.
+ Depending on the circumstances, highly trained first aiders may need to move the patient (with minimal movement to the spine) so that a spinal board may be used.
+ With assistance, roll the patient onto their side using a log roll, ensuring that the head and spine remain in a neutral position.
+ Gently position the spinal board against the patient's back in line with their spine, ensuring the neutral position is maintained.
+ With the spinal board remaining as close to the back as possible at all times, slowly roll the patient (and

spinal board) backwards so that the spinal board ends up lying flat underneath the patient's back in a horizontal position.
+ Secure and immobilise the patient using head blocks and patient straps around the body.
+ Offer constant reassurance to the patient during this process and keep them informed as to what you are doing. Being totally immobilised can be frightening and feeling anxious and panicked may make the patient try to struggle.
+ Monitor the patient's vital signs and condition until medical help arrives.

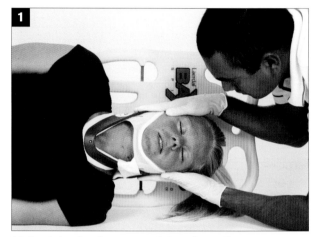

Maintaining head support while in log roll

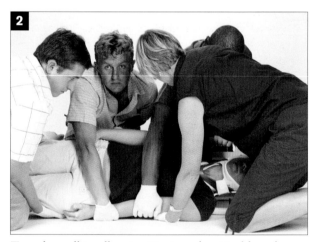

Team log roll to allow positioning of a spinal board

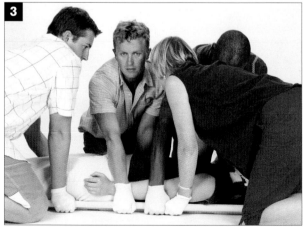

Team log roll to roll patient back to the horizontal position

for conscious, standing patients on land

The following technique is the preferred method for conscious and standing patients with a suspected spinal injury.

✚ If possible, maintain and support the head in the neutral position by placing hands either side of the patient's head.

✚ A cervical collar should be fitted and applied by trained personnel only.

✚ Size up a spinal board alongside the patient for the correct height.

✚ Insert the spinal board on an angle in between the patient's spine and the first aider's arms at the head, ensuring that the board is placed as close as possible to the patient's heels. Bring the board to the upright position between the first aider and the patient's back.

✚ If the patient feels faint while standing, lie them against the spinal board (see 'improvising if no straps are available' below).

✚ Apply head blocks to further immobilise the cervical spine and fasten the body straps across the patient, ensuring that straps across the chest do not constrict their breathing.

✚ Grasping the board at spaced positions, the first aiders slowly and smoothly lower the patient down to the ground. Before lowering the patient, it is recommended that a first aider place their feet at the base of the front of the spinal board to avoid it slipping while lowering the board into the horizontal position.

✚ When lowering the patient, all first aiders except the first aider at the head should be positioned so that they are facing the patient's head with the side of their body perpendicular to the long axis of the spinal board. This allows safe handling practices when lowering the patient.

✚ Offer constant reassurance to the patient during this process and keep them informed as to what you are doing.

✚ Monitor the patient's vital signs and condition until medical help arrives.

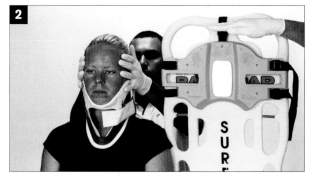

Sizing of spinal board to patient

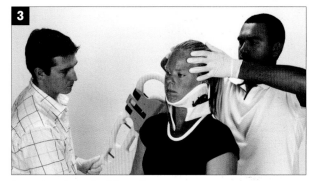

Inserting the spinal board

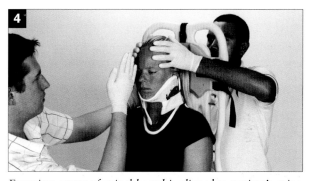

Ensuring centre of spinal board is aligned to patient's spine

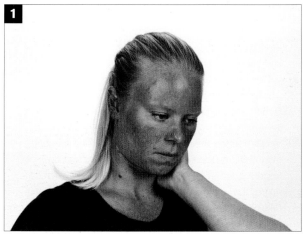

Patient indicating neck pain

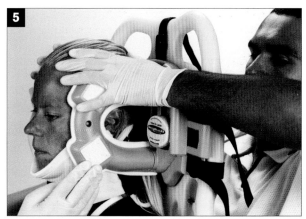

Application of headblocks (ensuring ears are free from pressure)

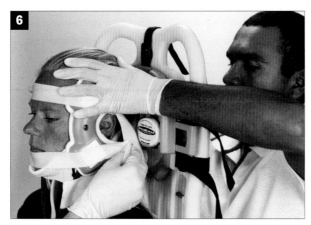

Application of forehead and chin straps

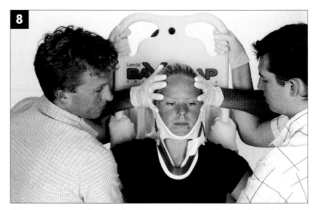

Insert arms under patient's armpits and hold the highest possible handle on the board

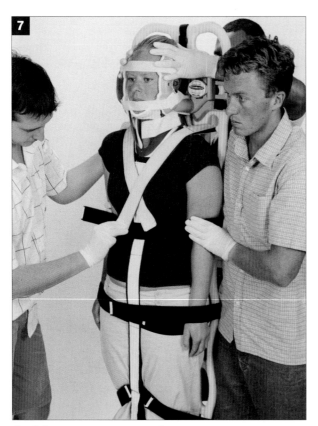

Applying straps to secure patient

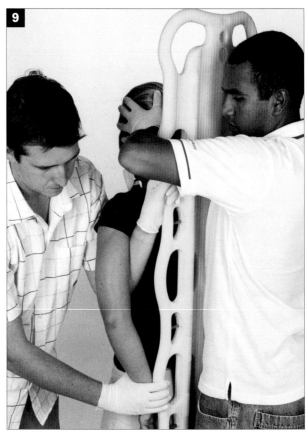

Secure patient's arm to spinal board

improvising if no straps are available

✚ If no straps are available, the assisting first aiders who placed the board into position should face the patient and each place one arm underneath the patient's armpits and grasp the highest hand hole possible on the spinal board. This position is designed to hold the patient's weight and temporarily secure them to the board.

✚ The first aiders should then grasp the top of the spinal board with their other arm ensuring that their arm is positioned underneath the first aider's arms stabilising the head.

✚ If extra assistance is required, bystanders should be asked to assist and placed at the top of the spinal board, beside the person stabilising the head, to assist in taking the primary weight of the patient. In this case, the first aiders holding the board under the patient's armpits should secure the patient's arms (one either side) to the board with their opposite hand.

✚ When the patient has been lowered to about 45 degrees, the first aider at the head will need to call "*stop*". All first aiders and bystanders maintain the patient in position while the first aider at the head slowly rotates their hands on the patient's head (maintaining pressure) to stabilise it, so that their fingers point in line with the patient's body.* Those taking the weight of the patient during lowering will take this time to readjust their positions to enable them to keep their backs vertical to lower the patient in the safest manner to meet manual handling requirements. When all are comfortably adjusted, the patient can be lowered to the horizontal position.

* In some circumstances with child patients, the first aider in control of the head may have to maintain head support by repositioning themselves in front of the spinal board rather than behind.

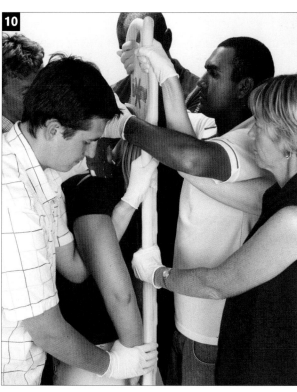

Remaining personnel inserting arms to assist with the lowering of the patient

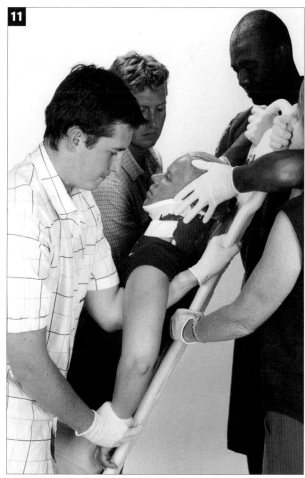

Gently lower the patient

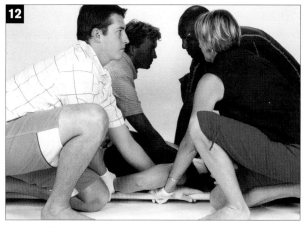

Lower the patient to the ground, maintaining a straight back

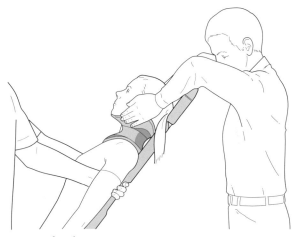

Maintain head support

for unconscious patients found floating in water

Many spinal injuries result from people diving into shallow water where rocks, sandbanks or foreign objects may be present. Spinal injuries in the aquatic environment have the added complication of possible drowning. Managing suspected spinal injuries in the aquatic environment is no different from on land — managing the patient's airway and breathing is the first priority while immobilising the body as much as possible. The preferred method for managing a spinal injury in the water is the extended arm roll over and the spinal stretcher carry.

✚ If a patient is found lying face down in shallow water, evaluate the scene and call for patient resources (e.g. extra first aiders, cervical collar and spinal board).

✚ Approaching the patient head on, reach underneath the patient's face and grasp their right upper arm (between the elbow and shoulder) with your right hand and the patient's left upper arm with your left hand. The arms should be grasped so that your thumbs point towards the feet of the patient with your fingers vertical.

✚ Holding the patient's arms in front of their body, immobilise the head by pressing their arms firmly against their head and neck.

✚ While moving backwards, slowly roll the patient so that their face (and airway) exits the water (by moving backwards the patient's body and feet will rise to the surface assisting in the roll).

✚ At this point, a second first aider should assist with a buoyant spinal board, which should be submerged under the patient and allowed to float up so that the centre of the board is in line with the patient's spine.

NOTE:
- In rough water conditions, the first aider should place their back to any oncoming waves to shield water from passing over the patient's face and airway.
- In white water environments first aiders need to observe the oncoming waves and swells vigilantly.
- Precautions have to be made to ensure that the arms maintain firm support of the head.

✚ If the patient is unconscious or in unstable waters, the patient must first be retrieved: lift them and carry from the water in a prompt manner. At all times, the patient should remain in the horizontal position and the head immobilised with the arms pressed firmly against the sides of their head. As many people as possible should be used to keep the patient's neck and spine aligned.

NOTE:
If the patient is conscious and in stable waters, cervical collars/immobilisation head blocks and straps should be applied (see spinal boards and head blocks).

✚ Leave the water under the direction of the first aider at the head of the patient. On reaching a stable environment, the patient should be lowered as carefully as possible, laying them flat on a safe surface. If the patient's cervical spine has not already been immobilised with a cervical collar or head blocks and straps, they should be applied promptly.

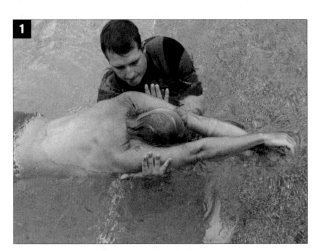

Grasping patient's arms and immobilising head

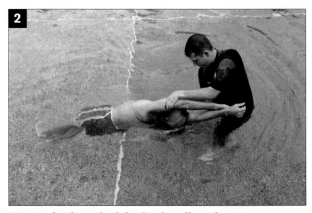

Moving backward while slowly rolling the patient

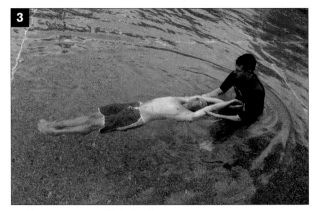

Roll patient onto their back

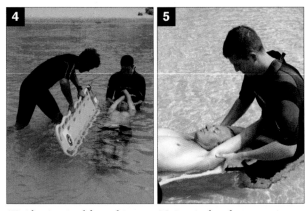

'Knifing' spinal board into position   *Maintain head support*

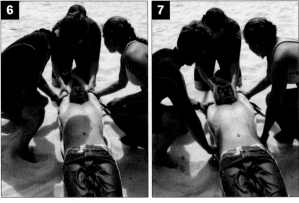

Immobilisation maintained while changing head support hand position

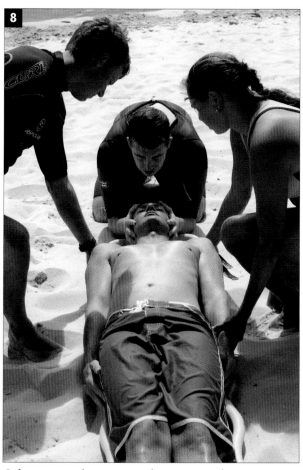

Other rescuers lower arms of patient together

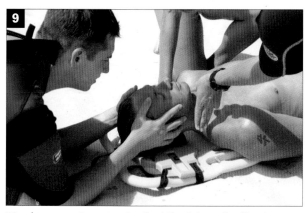

Head support is maintained while sizing of collar is measured

vice grip

Another form of spinal immobilisation in calm aquatic environments (e.g swimming pool, flat ocean, dam, etc) is the vice grip. This can be used in shallow or deep water. If the casualty is face down, a vice grip roll over can be used to move them into a face-up position, while maintaining immobilisation.

✚ Place the patient's arms beside their body.
✚ Approaching the patient from one side, reach under the patient and grip the patient's jaw with one hand, with your forearm lying directly over the sternum.
✚ Place your other hand on the back of the patient's head with your forearm lying along the patient's spine,

ensuring that the grip is supporting the head and spine without pressing on the soft tissues of the neck.
✚ Squeeze your forearms together to create a vice to support the head and neck.
✚ If the patient needs to be rolled into a face-up position, move under the casualty without lifting them out of the water (which may cause movement of the spine) to surface on the other side of the patient. Walking or swimming forwards during the roll will assist in elevating the patient's body and legs (an alternative technique should be used in very shallow water, where the first aider is unable to move under the patient).
✚ The rest of the retrieval should be performed as described above.
✚ The patient's vital signs and condition should be monitored until medical help arrives.

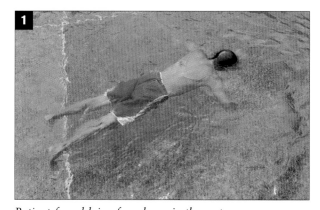

Patient found lying face down in the water

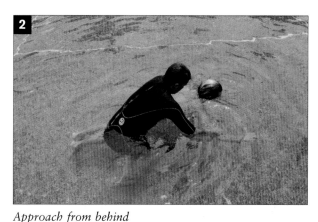

Approach from behind

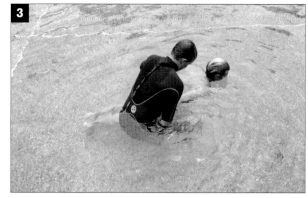

Move the patient's arms beside the body

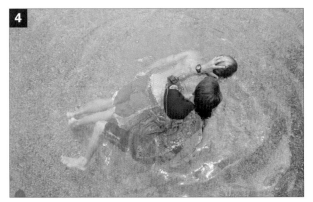

Place arms directly in line with the spine and sternum, supporting the head

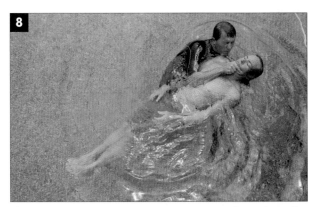

Monitor patient's condition after emerging from the roll

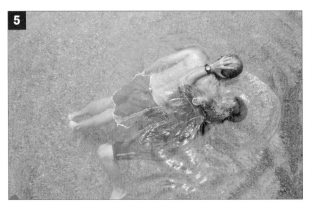

Roll under the patient

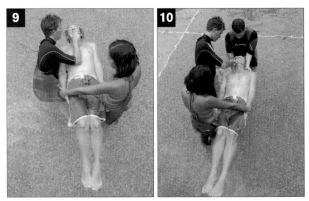

Second rescuer supporting the weight of the patient at the hips

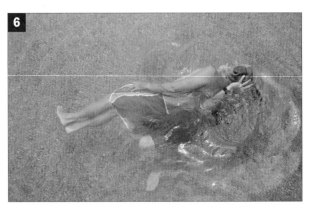

Maintain back and head support throughout the roll

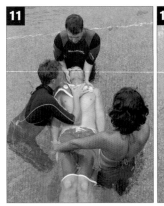

Application of cervical collar

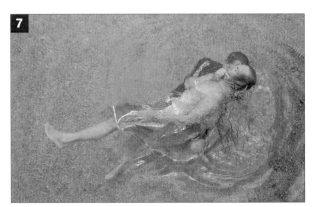

'As above'

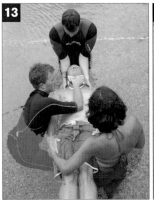

Reapply vice grip between patient and bottom of collar

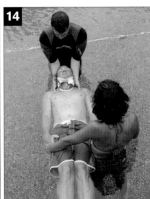

Third rescuer applies full head clamp

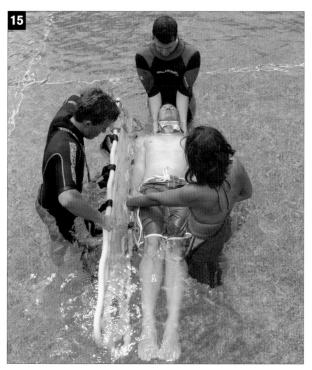

Spinal board 'knifed' under patient into position

transporting casualties

All patients with a suspected spinal injury should be transported to a hospital for further medical examination. Trained personnel should transport patients.

In some instances it may not be possible to move the patient, because of danger to the first aider and bystanders (i.e. surf environment, car explosion after accident).

Patients should only be transported if the following criteria have been met, unless the patient is not breathing and has no pulse:

+ unconscious
+ cervical collar applied
+ spinal board (or standard device) used with straps
+ head immobilised.

The patient should be transported in the horizontal position with the appropriate amount of first aiders assisting in the carry. However, this may not be possible in all circumstances, due to irregular obstacles.

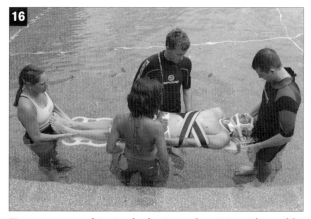

Transport casualties in the horizontal position, if possible

revision

1. Complete the following sentences about spinal injuries.

    With proper ………………, if the spinal cord has not been ……………… or damaged on the initial impact, it can be

    protected against further ……………….. Unless an accident has been ……………… or if a spinal injury is highly

    improbable, always treat motionless and ……………… patients for a spinal injury.

2. What are the two mechanisms operating in the majority of spinal injuries?

    a) _____   b) _____

3. List five symptoms of spinal injury:

    a) _____

    b) _____

    c) _____

    d) _____

    e) _____

4. Complete the following sentence about moving casualties with suspected spinal injuries.

    Casualties found lying in ……………… or unusual positions should not be ……………… unless under the

    supervision of an ……………… rescue and/or health care worker with specific ………………, unless they are at

    risk of ………………..

5. When moving casualties with suspected spinal injuries, what are the priorities in order of importance?

    a) _____

    b) _____

    c) _____

Answers appear in Appendix 8.

triage

learning outcomes

Perform triage in a multiple-casualty situation.

+ Describe the importance of triage for managing multiple patients.
+ Detail the approach to assessing a patient at a major incident.
+ Detail the approach to assessing multiple patients during triage.
+ Demonstrate the START triage system.

how you may be assessed

underpinning knowledge

A number of oral or written questions may be asked relating to the importance of triage, triage at major incidents, assessing multiple patients and the START triage system. Examples have been included at the end of the chapter.

practical demonstration

You may be asked to demonstrate how to assess multiple patients during triage. You may be asked to demonstrate the START triage system.

scenario

You may be required to perform triage on a number of patients with different injuries and first aid/emergency care needs.

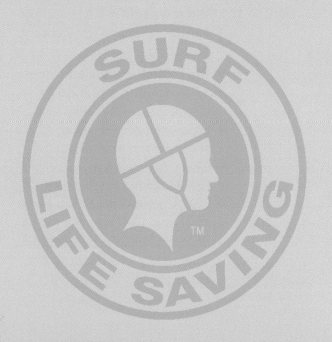

what is triage?

Triage is the initial assessment and sorting of patients based on medical need and likely response to treatment. In a multiple-casualty situation, triage is essential to effectively sort patients and prioritise their order of treatment to ensure that the greatest good can be done for as many patients as possible. Triage does not apply to a single patient, however the principles of assessment and management can be used to determine the degree of urgency in the management of most patients.

triage in action

Triage is essential for managing multiple-casualty events as it:

+ prioritises treatment to use available resources as efficiently as possible
+ ensures care is focused on those patients most likely to benefit from the limited resources available
+ provides a framework for difficult and stressful life-and-death decisions
+ creates order in a chaotic environment.

approach to a major incident

The following steps outline the procedure for systematically assessing a patient involved in a major incident.

approach to an incident

After notifying the appropriate authorities, (i.e. ambulance, fire, police) there are 6 steps in the approach to an incident:

1. **Is the area safe?**
   + Assess safety and, if necessary, control hazards.
2. **Is the patient alive/dead/in a life-threatening situation?**
   + Check the patient's response.
   + Ensure the patient has an adequate and clear airway.
   + Check for breathing.
   + Ensure adequate ventilation.
   + Check pulse — if cardiac arrest, administer CPR and defibrillation.
   + Ensure care of the cervical spine, if necessary, or if the patient is unconscious.

   + Control life-threatening haemorrhage.
3. **Is the patient 'time-critical'?**
   + Assess vital signs — perfusion status, respiratory status, state of consciousness.
   + Identify the main presenting problem — if trauma, establish the type of trauma (pattern of actual injury or illness) and what caused the injury (mechanism of injury).
   + Assess whether the patient is experiencing physiological distress ('actual time-critical') or, if not, whether the patient is likely to deteriorate without appropriate care ('emergent time-critical').
4. **Initial management.**
   + Ensure the patient is in the appropriate position.
   + Ensure the patient rests, and give reassurance.
   + Administer oxygen, if necessary, if a unit and qualified personnel are available.
5. **Perform a secondary assessment.**
6. **Continue management and monitoring of situation.**

Recognition of the 'time-critical' patient, providing appropriate care, and ensuring early notification of the ambulance service will improve patient management and ensure the best possible outcome for the patient.

assessing multiple patients

In multiple-casualty events, it will not be possible to fully assess and provide initial treatment to all patients as outlined above. Invariably, some patients will be more severely injured and, in the absence of qualified medical personnel, it is the unenviable role of the most experienced first aider to assess and prioritise treatment.

Initial assessment should be guided by the above steps, though, based on the number of patients involved, there may be no time to take vital signs or treat injuries at this stage. A good impression of the severity of a patient's injuries can be made from the presenting problem and general appearance of the patient. The triage assessment should only take a few minutes so all patients can be assessed before prioritising. Triage should be prioritised over treatment and only the following procedures should be carried out while assessing patients:

+ ensure the airway is open
+ control major bleeds
+ elevate the legs.

START

The START triage system (**S**imple **T**reatment **A**nd **R**apid Treatment) classifies a patient's treatment category from an assessment of their respiratory (respiratory rate), circulatory (capillary refill) and neurological function (ability to obey simple commands). Patients are then attributed to one of the following four categories.

1. *Immediate (red tag):* patients with life-threatening but treatable injuries requiring immediate medical attention are assigned a red tag. These patients are the first to be transported to hospital when medical help arrives, without delaying transportation for stabilisation.
2. *Urgent (orange tag):* patients with serious injuries, but able to wait a short time for treatment are assigned an orange tag.
3. *Delayed (green tag):* patients who can wait hours to days for treatment are assigned a green tag. These patients can be separated from the more seriously injured by asking for patients able to walk (i.e. 'minor' patients) to congregate in a specified area.
4. *Dead (white or black tag):* patients who are dead or not expected to live because of the severity of their injuries and the limited resources available. These patients are assigned either a white or black tag.

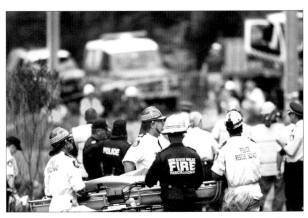

At disaster and accident scenes, triage can save lives by prioritising serious injuries

Tragically, in the event of a major incident, patients in cardiac or respiratory arrest who require lengthy EAR and/or CPR, often to no avail, should only be resuscitated if there are no other life-threatening or imminently life-threatening injuries that require urgent attention. Similarly, pre-existing disease and age should be factored into triage decisions. Objectivity is critical for triage to ensure a good outcome for as many people as possible.

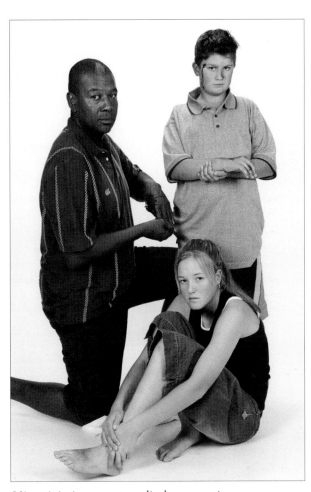

Minor injuries are not medical emergencies

NOTE:
- Save life over limb.
- Do not move patients before triage unless absolutely necessary.
- Never delay transportation to stabilise 'immediate' casualties.
- Casualties with minor injuries may be able to assist in the management of critical casualties.

revision

1. Define triage.

_____

_____

2. List four reasons why triage is essential for managing multiple-casualty events.

    a) _____

    b) _____

    c) _____

    d) _____

3. What are the only procedures that should be carried out while assessing patients?

    a) _____   b) _____   c) _____

4. Define 'immediate' patients according to the START triage system.

    _____

    _____

5. Define 'delayed' patients according to the START triage system.

    _____

    _____

6. Define 'minor' patients according to the START triage system.

    _____

    _____

7. Define and describe the START triage system.

    _____

    _____

    _____

    _____

Answers appear in Appendix 8.

advanced resuscitation and oxygen administration

learning outcomes

Perform advanced resuscitation techniques and administer oxygen during first aid and emergency care.

+ Describe why oxygen may be used in first aid and emergency care.
+ Detail the safety precautions to be observed by first aiders when using oxygen.
+ Describe the components of oxygen resuscitation equipment.
+ Demonstrate the routine checks of oxygen resuscitation equipment.
+ Demonstrate how to administer oxygen therapy.
+ Demonstrate the setting up of oxygen resuscitation equipment.
+ Detail the maintenance of oxygen resuscitation equipment.
+ Detail the procedure for administering suction.
+ Detail the procedure for administering oxygen using an automatic oxygen-powered resuscitator.
+ Detail the care and use of oropharyngeal airways.

See Appendix 7 for the safe handling of medical gases

how you may be assessed

underpinning knowledge

A number of oral or written questions may be asked relating to the use of oxygen, safety precautions, oxygen resuscitation equipment, routine checks, setting up equipment, administering oxygen, maintenance of equipment, suction, automatic oxygen-powered resuscitators and oropharyngeal airways. Examples have been included at the end of the chapter.

practical demonstration

You may be asked to demonstrate the routine checks of oxygen resuscitation equipment. You may be asked to demonstrate the administration of oxygen therapy. You may be asked to demonstrate the setting up of oxygen resuscitation equipment.

scenario

You may be required to use oxygen on one or more patients who require oxygen therapy or resuscitation.

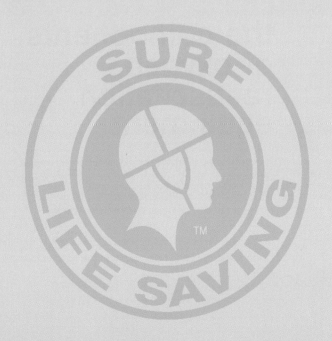

why use oxygen?

Oxygen administration is useful for any patient who does not appear to be adequately perfused or not maintaining sufficient oxygen levels. Qualified personnel may safely administer oxygen to any patient who is not adequately perfused. Patients likely to benefit from oxygen include those with the following conditions:

+ unconsciousness
+ shock
+ blood loss
+ chest pain
+ shortness of breath, including asthma
+ circulatory distress
+ severe pain
+ injuries
+ after resuscitation
+ absent breathing.

safety precautions when using oxygen

Oxygen must be used with care and respect at all times.

+ Never use oxygen near an open flame.
+ Never use oxygen near cigarettes.
+ Never use grease or oil with oxygen equipment.
+ Remember that oxygen promotes all types of burning (combustion).
+ Do not allow anyone to tamper with oxygen equipment.
+ Store the oxygen unit in a cool place.
+ Store oxygen bottles lying flat, or securely fastened, if upright.
+ Use only medical oxygen.
+ Never use oxygen when delivering a shock via a defibrillator.

the components of oxygen resuscitation equipment

It is very important for those trained in the use of oxygen resuscitation units to ensure that they are familiar with the components and operation of the unit(s) in use at their location. The basic components are listed.

+ *Protective case:* This houses all the relevant equipment. In some models, it incorporates the oxygen cylinder itself.

+ *Medical oxygen cylinder:* The body of the cylinder is usually black or silver/grey and the shoulders of oxygen cylinders are white (it may also come in a silver cylinder marked 'medical oxygen'). Note that medical oxygen is the only gas to be used in the oxygen equipment. The cylinder has two pin index holes next to the main outlet. These index holes mate with pins on the mounting yoke of the oxygen equipment. A fresh, full cylinder will usually have a protective wrapping of blue or white plastic around the oxygen outlet to prevent dust and dirt from entering during transport. Before attaching the cylinder to the oxygen equipment, all wrapping must be removed and the cylinder 'cracked' by quickly and gently opening and closing the outlet valve.
+ *Cylinder cradle:* This provides support for the oxygen cylinder.
+ *Cylinder yoke:* This is the connection for the oxygen cylinder. In some instances, it is part of the case; otherwise, it may be attached as part of the regulator.
+ *Sealing washer (Bodock sealer):* This fits in the yoke to prevent leakage from the cylinder joint. Spare seals are kept in the oxygen equipment case.
+ *Locating pins:* These are positioned in the yoke, so that the operator can locate the oxygen cylinder correctly.
+ *Thumb screw:* This helps to secure and maintain the cylinder in position.
+ *Cylinder key wheel:* This is used to open or close the cylinder valve.
+ *External cylinder connection:* This allows larger oxygen cylinders to be attached. It is important to remember that when an external cylinder is in use, a small cylinder or the yoke plug should be firmly in place to prevent oxygen leaking. This connection is not found on all units.
+ *Contents gauge:* This indicates the amount of oxygen in the cylinder.
+ *Regulator:* This regulates the oxygen pressure and flow of oxygen to the therapy and oxygen control valve(s).
+ *OP airways:* Oropharyngeal airways help maintain a clear airway and should be used only by trained personnel.
+ *Airbag:* This silicone-based apparatus is used for inflating a patient's lungs by squeezing, which supplies oxygen from an oxygen reservoir bag.
+ *Oxygen reservoir bag:* Attached to the airbag.
+ *Tubing:* Depending on the unit, there will be either one or two tubes, usually clear and/or green in colour.
+ *Control valves:* These are turned on when using the airbag resuscitator or oxygen therapy, giving a fixed flow rate of oxygen. On some models, the control valve and flow rate are built into the regulator.
+ *Anaesthetic masks:* Each unit should contain at least one adult and at least one child-sized mask.
+ *Therapy masks:* Each unit contains at least one adult and child-sized mask. A clear, colourless, disposable type of therapy mask is recommended.
+ *Chalk:* This is used to mark the volume of oxygen in the cylinder.
+ *Gloves:* Used for personal protection.
+ *Pens, pencils and paper:* Used for taking records during oxygen usage.

other equipment

+ *Automatic oxygen-powered resuscitator:* These devices deliver oxygen under high pressure to inflate the lungs of patients who are not breathing.
+ *Suction:* This feature helps the operator to remove fluids from the patient's mouth.

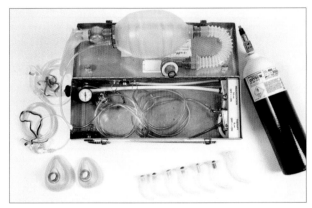

An Oxyviva unit

NOTE:
The SLSA Oxygen Equipment Policy is located on the SLSA website at www.slsa.asn.au.

routine check of equipment

+ Before a cylinder is fitted to the oxygen equipment, remove the protective plastic wrapping.
+ 'Crack' the cylinder by turning it on and off very briefly, keeping it as upright as possible and taking care that the outlet is not pointed at any person or potential danger (e.g. sand). Cracking the cylinder removes any foreign matter from its valve opening.
+ The cylinder must be inserted into the yoke, lining up the inlet and outlet holes together with the locating pins and spigot.
+ Check that the sealing washer is present and is not damaged or dirty, otherwise the equipment is inoperable and cannot be used. Then, firmly screw home the thumb screw.
+ Check the contents of the cylinder by using the key wheel to open the cylinder valve slowly until the gauge reaches a steady point. This slow build-up of pressure saves damage to the regulator and gauge, which can occur from a sudden rush of pressure. Open the cylinder valves fully, then turn the key wheel back half a turn to prevent locking. The gauge should register 'full'. Reject the cylinder if it is half or less than half full, and fit a new cylinder.
+ Check the oxygen tubing for cracks or other damage. Ensure that the open end will fit easily to both therapy masks.
+ Check both therapy masks for cleanliness and serviceability.
+ Check the condition of the anaesthetic mask cuffs for fit, perishing or cracks.

+ Ensure the oropharyngeal airways are present and clean. These are for use by appropriately qualified personnel.
+ Check in the case for:
  — *chalk* for marking the amount of oxygen in the cylinder
  — *pens, pencils and paper* for keeping records
  — *gloves* for personal protection during emergency care
  — *spare sealing washers* to replace defective or missing seals, as required.
+ Check the flow of oxygen from the cylinder through the tubing.
+ Check that there is no odour from the oxygen being expelled from the tubing.
+ Check the clear, colourless and green oxygen tubing for cracks or other damage, and ensure that the open end of the tube is fitted to the oxygen intake port of the airbag or therapy mask.
+ Check the operation of the oxygen nipples by turning the oxygen valves to the 'on' position. When you do this, oxygen should come out of both the therapy mask and oxygen tubing.
+ Check the airbag.
+ Close the cylinder valve, then drain oxygen from the system by operating both delivery systems. Check that the needle on the oxygen cylinder's contents gauge falls to zero.
+ Keep the whole unit clean and free from sand, sea water, oil and grease.
+ Check additional equipment (e.g. suction, automatic oxygen-powered resuscitators).

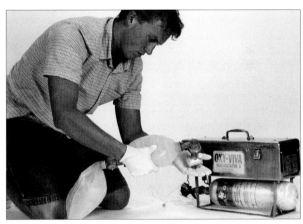

Checking oxygen equipment

suction

+ Remove large suction tubing from the case and hold near open end.
+ Turn suction lever fully on.
+ Test for suction against a soft part of one hand (tube should attach to the hand).
+ Turn lever off.
+ Remove catheter and fit to large tubing.
+ Turn suction lever fully on.
+ Test for suction again.
+ Turn lever off.
+ Return to case in original position.

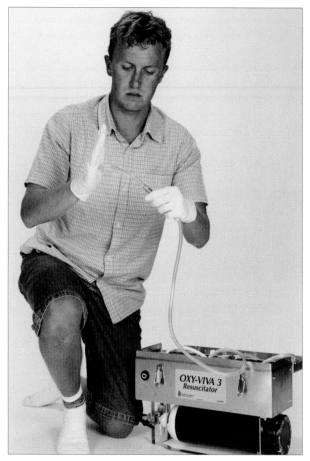

Suction checks

automatic oxygen-powered resuscitator

As per oxygen equipment plus:

✚ Block off the powerhead/demand valve outlet with one hand and trigger the device.
— Check for valve release.
— Check for blockages.

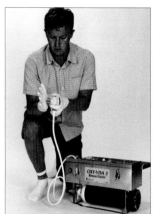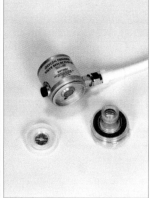

Powerhead checks

 NOTE:
As each item is checked, it should be returned to the case in a neat and tidy fashion.

administering oxygen therapy

✚ Check oxygen equipment before each use.
✚ When oxygen is in use, the equipment must be placed so that the operator responsible for it can reach it easily and can see the contents gauge.
✚ Connect the therapy mask to the tubing and turn on the oxygen. You should be able to feel and hear the oxygen coming through the mask.
✚ Put the mask on the patient's face ensuring it is secure by adjusting the elastic and pinching the metal noseband. Reassure the patient and inform them about what you are doing.

NOTE:
If a conscious patient does not want to use the mask, they can hold the mask in front of their face, or remove the tubing from it and direct the oxygen flow around the mouth and nose.

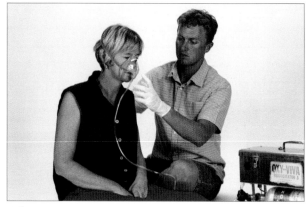

Administering oxygen

mouth-to-mask resuscitation with oxygen

Research has shown that adding oxygen during mouth-to-mask resuscitation can increase the oxygen received by the patient from 16% to 50% (16% is the oxygen content of expired air). If the therapy setting of 8 L per

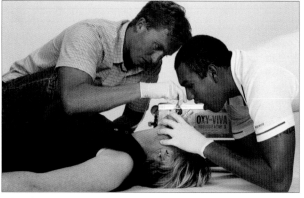

Mouth-to-mask resuscitation with supplemental oxygen

minute is used, the concentration of oxygen in the patient's lungs will be almost 45%, but if the resuscitation setting of 14–15 L per minute is used and the seal is good, the concentration for the patient will be greater (i.e. >50%). It is recommended that the higher setting be used if there is enough oxygen available for the time resuscitation is expected to last. If not, the flow of 8 litres per minute is satisfactory.

A number of different facemasks are approved for use in mouth-to-mask resuscitation. Some of these have oxygen ports that allow the oxygen therapy tubing to be connected.

Mouth-to-mask resuscitation with oxygen can be a one-operator operation, however, it is preferable that two operators are used. One person needs to do mouth-to-mask resuscitation while a second person handles the oxygen unit. The oxygen is turned to the appropriate setting and the tubing fitted either to the oxygen port, through the opening of the mask, or through the cheek of the mask if an adequate seal is maintained. Masks with ports are highly recommended for this procedure.

Airbag checks

✚ Check the airbag for leaks and direction of airflow by blocking the patient valve with the thumb or hand and compressing the bag under reasonable pressure. The air should not leak out of the rear valve, the bag or the patient valve. Then release the thumb or hand, whereupon the bag should compress and refill rapidly.

✚ Check the function of the yellow disc membrane on the patient valve. Place the oxygen reservoir bag over the patient valve and inflate it fully by squeezing the ventilation bag. Then squeeze the reservoir bag gently and the yellow disc membrane will lift. During resuscitation, the patient exhales through this disc membrane.

✚ Check the overflow membrane of the reservoir valve (Laerdal bag only). Inflate the reservoir bag as before and connect it to the reservoir valve. Compress the reservoir bag rapidly and watch the yellow-seated disc lift. This membrane ensures that the reservoir bag cannot be overfilled with oxygen.

✚ The air-intake membrane is located in the rear valve of the airbag and the reservoir valve of the Laerdal bag. Check its function by inflating the reservoir bag as before and connecting it to the airbag. With continued compressions of the ventilation bag, the reservoir bag will empty and the ventilation bag will draw in air through the air-intake membrane.

airbag oxygen resuscitator

The airbag resuscitator with oxygen reservoir is a manually operated, soft-recoil silicone bag with a secondary plastic bag attached. This secondary plastic bag acts as a reservoir for oxygen when connected to an external oxygen supply.

The resuscitator with oxygen reservoir will supply the patient with up to 95% oxygen when connected to an oxygen supply, with a flow rate of 14–15 L per minute.

Patients who are not breathing should be treated initially using EAR, but they will almost always benefit from the administration of supplemental oxygen by trained personnel.

When the oxygen unit arrives and is being set up, the first operator should continue with the mouth-to-mask resuscitation method (or change to it, if a mask was not previously available) while preparing to change over to the bag. This may take some time, however, and resuscitation must continue during the changeover period. It is possible to give mouth-to-mask resuscitation with oxygen briefly using the therapy tubing before the bag is ready, as there are two separate tubes.

setting up oxygen resuscitation equipment

✚ The oxygen equipment operator needs to inform others about who they are and their qualifications to operate the equipment.

✚ The oxygen equipment operator sets up the machine clear of the patient and both operators, but in a position where the pressure gauge is clearly visible.

✚ Immediately upon opening the case, a suitably sized anaesthetic mask is passed to the EAR operator to change to the mouth-to-mask resuscitation method. If mouth-to-mask resuscitation is in progress, however, the airbag oxygen resuscitator can be fitted directly to the mask (after an operational check).

✚ The oxygen equipment operator should quickly check:
   — the correct operation of the patient valve
   — the valve to the oxygen reservoir bag
   — the connection to the oxygen supply.

✚ The oxygen is then turned on to 14–15 L per minute to allow inflation of the airbag reservoir.

procedure

✚ When the oxygen reservoir is inflated, the oxygen equipment operator tells the other operator that the airbag is ready for use.

✚ After a signal — usually the equipment operator taps the other operator on the shoulder and explains what they are about to do — the equipment operator positions the patient valve in the anaesthetic mask and compresses the airbag so that there is no change at all in the timing of respiratory resuscitation, which is important if CPR is being performed.

✚ The airbag oxygen resuscitator should be compressed with two hands (for an adult) using a gentle squeezing motion, taking at least 1.5–2 seconds for the chest to rise.

✚ The amount of oxygen to be squeezed into the patient's chest is the amount required to make the chest rise. The bag should then be released and allowed to refill.

NOTE:
The rise and fall of the patient's chest should be watched at all times during this procedure.

From this stage on, the procedure for the use of oxygen equipment is identical to that for EAR (see Chapter 4).

+ On the changeover to the oxygen equipment, the EAR operator controls the backward head tilt and ensures a proper seal between the mask and the patient's face. Meanwhile, the oxygen equipment operator manages the airbag and oxygen system.
+ Both operators are responsible for seeing that the patient's chest rises with each inflation and falls as air exits the lungs.
+ If, at any time, either operator is not happy with the functioning of the oxygen equipment, the equipment must be removed immediately and EAR must continue by the mouth-to-mouth, mouth-to-mask or mouth-to-nose method.
+ If the airbag oxygen resuscitator is being used during CPR, at least two operators must be present, although it is highly recommended that three rescuers be present. One controls the patient's airway and ensures the seal of the anaesthetic mask; the second activates the oxygen equipment; and the third performs ECC. If only two operators are present, one should control the airway, ensure the mask seal and activate the oxygen equipment while the second operator conducts ECC.
+ If oxygen equipment is being used on a child, the paediatric airbag (if available) should be used and compressed with one hand. When the child's chest is seen to rise, stop compression of the bag. Airbag resuscitators not specifically manufactured for the exclusive use on infants should not be used on infants.
+ If the oxygen bottle is depleted during resuscitation, continue to use the airbag resuscitator equipment and remove the reservoir bag.

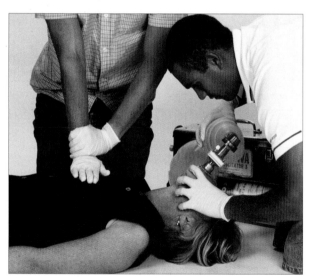

CPR with oxygen

operational time

A full 'C' cylinder (440–490 L) will have the following approximate operational times:

+ 50 minutes, with continuous use of oxygen therapy at ~8 L per minute

+ 30 minutes, with continuous use of airbag (and oxygen) at ~14–15 L per minute.

equipment maintenance
general care

+ The machine should be kept clean and free of sand and foreign materials.
+ To ensure its correct operation, equipment must be checked:
    — after every teaching session
    — before use each day.
+ Whenever the oxygen equipment shows defects that may cause it to operate incorrectly, the machine must be taken out of service immediately and repaired by the manufacturer.
+ The oxygen equipment should be serviced at least every 12 months, or according to the manufacturer's recommendations.

care after use

After every use, the resuscitator should be disassembled, cleaned, disinfected, reassembled and tested in an orderly sequence.

 NOTE:
When using the Laerdal bag, do not remove the plastic adaptor from the patient end of the airbag or the reusable reservoir.

+ Oxygen therapy masks should be sent to hospital with the patient or disposed of after use.
+ The tube and the anaesthetic masks should be washed thoroughly in warm soapy water so that all foreign material is removed, then rinsed with fresh running water.
+ The patient valve and the rear valve should be disassembled, washed in warm soapy water, then rinsed in fresh running water and reassembled.
+ The airbag should be washed in warm soapy water and rinsed in fresh running water.
+ The reservoir valve (on the Laerdal bag) and oxygen reservoir should be washed in warm soapy water and rinsed in fresh running water.
+ All contaminated parts should be soaked in a solution of 70% alcoholic chlorhexidine or a hypochlorite solution (bleach) for at least 2 minutes, then rinsed and dried.
+ Operate all parts of the equipment after drying and before storage to ensure that the equipment is ready for use the next time it is needed.

storage

✚ Store oxygen equipment in a cool, but accessible place, as heat causes rubber and plastic components to deteriorate.

✚ Spare oxygen cylinders should be stored near the oxygen equipment.

✚ Store oxygen equipment away from busy traffic areas and sand and dust contamination.

✚ Do not store oxygen equipment near oil or grease — these substances can cause fire when in contact with high-pressure oxygen.

✚ Do not store the equipment in an enclosed space or cover it over — any leakage from the unit could cause oxygen build-up, which is dangerous in the event of fire.

✚ Do not allow smoking or naked flames near the oxygen equipment at any time, whether it is stored or in use. Leaking oxygen can fuel a fire.

✚ Do not leave the unit with any pressure in the system. Turn off the cylinder, then drain the oxygen from the delivery tubes by operating either of the two delivery systems.

✚ Return empty oxygen cylinders for filling without delay. Cylinders that are half-full or less can be used for training.

administering suction (optional)

Types of suction devices include:

✚ electric — use in first aid room
✚ foot pump — use outdoors
✚ vacuum bottle
✚ hand pump.

The principles of use are similar for all types.

procedure

✚ Suction is only used in an unconscious patient or a semiconscious patient, where they cannot cough or swallow.

✚ Wearing gloves, the suction catheter is removed from its sterile packaging and attached to the suction tubing.

✚ Measure the distance from the centre of the lips to the angle of the jaw and place your fingers that distance from the catheter tip. Ensure the catheter does not extend past the back of the patient's teeth.

✚ Lubricate the catheter by dipping it in saline or the patient's saliva.

✚ Open the mouth.

✚ Suction may be repeated several times but for no longer than 15 seconds before it is removed and washed in saline. This prevents hypoxia developing, as suction will also reduce air available to the lungs.

✚ Make sure that the area between the teeth and the cheek is also sucked out as well as under the tongue.

If the patient is conscious then the suction tip will cause a gag reflex. In this case suction is probably not needed, as the patient is unlikely to have a compromised airway, as they will also have a swallow reflex.

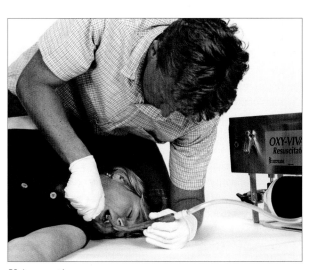

Using suction

 NOTE:
Oxygen-driven suction consumes considerable oxygen (20–40 L/min). It is essential that you close the valve immediately after use.

automatic oxygen-powered resuscitator (optional)

Manually triggered oxygen-powered ventilators deliver positive pressure enabling a non-breathing patient to be ventilated with 100% oxygen. Most of these devices incorporate a demand valve, which will provide inspired oxygen levels of 100% to a breathing patient.

Warning: There is an increased risk of distension of the stomach in the patient who does not have a cuffed endo-tracheal tube in place. There is also an increased risk of over-inflation of the lungs and damage to the middle ear due to changes in barometric pressure (barotrauma) in the patient who is intubated. This technique should only be used by competent regular users of this equipment.

procedure

✚ Oxygen supply is turned on.
✚ If necessary, the control lever or equivalent is turned to 'on', 'automatic' or whatever is appropriate to start automatic function.
✚ If the resuscitator has a tidal flow and/or frequency control, these are adjusted.

+ Clear the airway (see Chapter 4) or use suction.
+ Open the airway using the head tilt/jaw support technique.
+ If accredited to do so, the operator may choose to insert the appropriate oropharyngeal airway.
+ Place the mask on the face, beginning at the bridge of the nose and then firmly over the rest of the face.
+ Hold the mask in position by placing one hand on either side of the mask with the index fingers over the lower half of the mask, the thumbs beside the bridge of the nose and two or three fingers under the jaw. Also use head tilt and jaw thrust.
+ Ensure adequate tidal volume is being delivered by observing the rise and fall of the chest. The tidal volume or frequency controls may require adjustment to achieve adequate ventilation.
+ For a patient who is breathing spontaneously, the control level or equivalent is changed to 'spontaneous' or its equivalent. Listen for the flow of oxygen into the device.

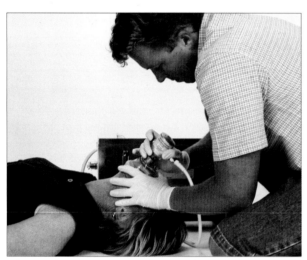

Using an automatic oxygen-powered resuscitator

oropharyngeal airways

Oropharyngeal (OP) airways are curved plastic devices that help keep the airway clear in the unconscious patient by depressing the tongue and keeping the teeth and lips apart. The OP airway by itself does not replace correct airway management practices and should be considered only as a tool to help in the management of a patient's airway.

An OP airway is a plastic device consisting of a rigid flange and a hollow curved tube. The flange, when

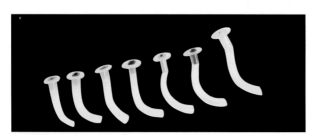

A set of OP airways

properly fitted, rests against the patient's lips. This flange does not prevent attaining an adequate seal from a facemask.

OP airways come in various sizes for different-sized patients. The smallest OP airways are approximately 5 cm long and the largest are over 10 cm in length.

OP airways are inserted using the 'rotation' method. This method is not recommended for infants or children under the age of 8 years.

care of OP airways

OP airways must be stored in a sterile state, preferably in a clear plastic bag. They should be easily accessible in the first aid kit, oxygen unit and first aid rooms.

OP airways should be checked for deformities such as cracks and scratches. Any damaged airway should be disposed of or used for training purposes only. Airways that are used specifically for training purposes should be marked 'Training use only'.

After training use, the OP airway should be washed in warm soapy water for at least 2 minutes. It should then be rinsed and dried and stored separately in a small, clean, clear plastic bag ready for use.

After use on a patient, the contaminated OP airway should be disposed of in a safe manner, preferably in an infectious-waste bag provided by attending ambulance or medical personnel. If this is not possible, the contaminated OP airway should be placed in an infectious-waste bag and stored in a safe place until proper disposal can be organised — usually through the local hospital.

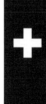

NOTE: Personal protection
* The prevalence of strains of hepatitis and HIV infection in the community has highlighted the need for great care when performing first aid or resuscitation. First aiders must avoid direct contact with the blood and other body substances of the person being treated.
* For first aiders' own safety, it is *strongly* recommended that they wear protective gloves and use a resuscitation mask for every first aid or resuscitation case.

choosing the appropriate-sized OP airway

To choose an OP airway of the correct size, place the airway against the side of the patient's face. The flange (top flattened end) of the airway will extend just past the centre of the patient's lips. The curve of the airway is then run sideways along the patient's jaw. The correct size airway is the one that reaches the angle of the patient's jaw.

when to insert an OP airway

The use of an OP airway is optional. First aiders should take less than 15 seconds to correctly size and insert an OP airway into a patient's mouth. Whether an OP airway

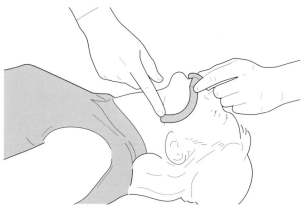

Sizing up for an OP airway using the distance from the lips to the angle of the jaw

is used or not, the management principles of DRABCD (see Chapter 3) do not change.

Ideally, the OP airway should be inserted into an unconscious patient's mouth after the patient has been rolled onto their side and their airway cleared.

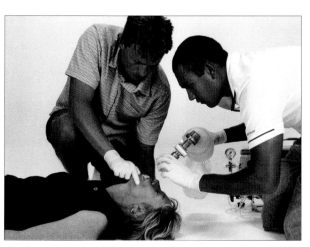

Applying a resuscitation mask over an OP airway

The airway can also be inserted during EAR or CPR while the patient is on their back. In this case, stop CPR or EAR and quickly insert the airway before continuing resuscitation. While the airway is being inserted, use the time to check the patient's pulse and/or call for assistance.

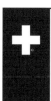

NOTE:
The OP airway should not be inserted during the delivery of external cardiac compressions, as this may impede the successful insertion of the airway and cause unnecessary injury to the patient.

inserting an OP airway

It is important to remember that OP airways must be inserted only into deeply unconscious or non-breathing patients. Insertion of an airway into a conscious patient may induce vomiting or gagging.

The OP airway should be inserted into the unconscious *breathing* patient in the lateral position. When a

patient is *not* breathing, the OP airway can be inserted with the patient on their side or back.

NOTE:
OP airways must be inserted *only* into deeply unconscious or non-breathing patients.

- Tilt the patient's head backwards; open the patient's mouth with one hand using jaw support or jaw thrust, if necessary (see Chapter 4).
- Visually check the patient's airway, and manually clear it, if necessary.
- Measure and choose an OP airway of the correct size.
- Remove the OP airway from the packet and lubricate it using moisture from the lips of the patient or with water.
- Hold the OP airway by the flange. With the tip pointing upwards towards the roof of the patient's mouth, insert the airway to approximately one-third of its length.

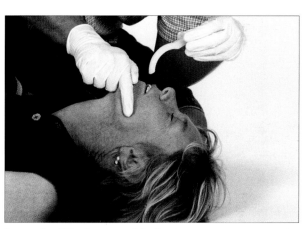

Insert the OP airway upside down

- When one-third of the airway is inside the mouth, rotate it 180° until the tip points downwards, at the same time sliding it over the patient's tongue in one smooth movement into the back of the pharynx until the flange is touching the lips.
- It should slip easily into place. If it is difficult, stop and reposition the patient's lower jaw and tongue before trying again. Never force it into position. Care is needed to avoid damage to the mouth and throat.

NOTE: Precautions when inserting an OP airway
- Ensure the lower lip is not pinched between the patient's teeth and the OP airway.
- Ensure that the OP airway does not push the tongue backwards and block the patient's airway.
- Ensure that you have adequate head tilt before inserting the OP airway.
- Don't force the OP airway into the mouth — it should slide in easily.

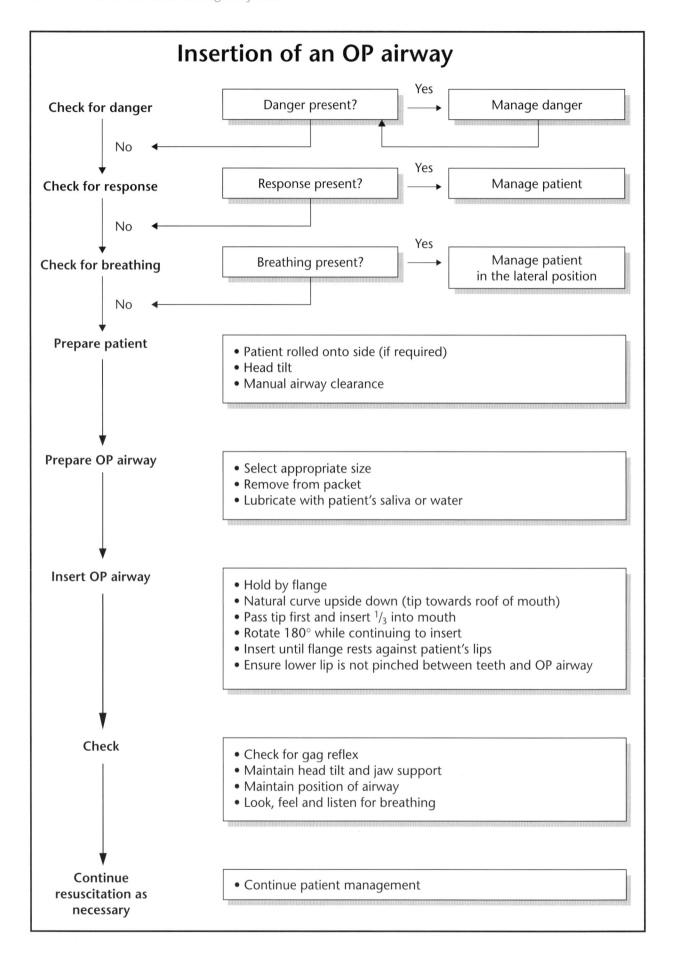

Insertion of an OP airway

Check for danger

Danger present? — Yes → Manage danger

No

Check for response

Response present? — Yes → Manage patient

No

Check for breathing

Breathing present? — Yes → Manage patient in the lateral position

No

Prepare patient

- Patient rolled onto side (if required)
- Head tilt
- Manual airway clearance

Prepare OP airway

- Select appropriate size
- Remove from packet
- Lubricate with patient's saliva or water

Insert OP airway

- Hold by flange
- Natural curve upside down (tip towards roof of mouth)
- Pass tip first and insert $1/3$ into mouth
- Rotate 180° while continuing to insert
- Insert until flange rests against patient's lips
- Ensure lower lip is not pinched between teeth and OP airway

Check

- Check for gag reflex
- Maintain head tilt and jaw support
- Maintain position of airway
- Look, feel and listen for breathing

Continue resuscitation as necessary

- Continue patient management

removing the OP airway

If the patient shows any signs of rejecting the OP airway, remove it immediately. In many cases, the patient may spit it out. The airway can be removed easily by sliding it out of the mouth following its natural curve.

NOTE:
Do not attempt to rotate the airway on removal. It is unnecessary and may cause damage to the mouth and pharynx.

important

OP airways should not be used:

✚ if the patient is conscious or semiconscious
— insertion of an OP airway into a conscious patient may induce vomiting or gagging
✚ if an airway of the correct size is not available
✚ if there is a large amount of vomit.

revision

1. List five conditions that may benefit from supplemental oxygen:

   a) _____   b) _____   c) _____

   d) _____   e) _____

2. Which of the following statements about safety precautions when using oxygen is *not* true?
   a) Never use oxygen near an open flame (including cigarettes).
   b) Never use grease or oil with oxygen equipment.
   c) When delivering a shock via defibrillator, make sure an oxygen mask is used.
   d) None of the above.

3. Complete the following information about oxygen therapy:

   A full 'C' cylinder (.................L) will have the following approximate operational times:
   • .... minutes, with continuous use of oxygen therapy at ~8 L per minute
   • 30 minutes, with continuous use of airbag (and oxygen) at ~................. L per minute.

4. What is an oropharyngeal (OP) airway?

   _____

   _____

5. What measurement is used to select the correct sized OP airway?

   _____

   _____

6. When shouldn't you use an OP airway?
   a) When the patient is conscious or semiconscious.
   b) When an airway of the correct size is not available.
   c) When there is a large amount of vomit.
   d) All of the above.

Answers appear in Appendix 8.

defibrillation

learning outcomes

Perform defibrillation during first aid and emergency care.

+ Describe what defibrillation is.
+ Detail the functions of a semi-automatic external defibrillator.
+ Detail the role of electrocardiograms during defibrillation.
+ Detail cardiac rhythm and arrhythmias during defibrillation.
+ Detail the types of semi-automatic external defibrillators.
+ Detail the defibrillation process using a semi-automatic external defibrillator.
+ Demonstrate the operation of a semi-automatic external defibrillator.
+ Detail the items kept with a semi-automatic defibrillator.
+ Detail the safety considerations for operators using a semi-automatic external defibrillator.

how you may be assessed

underpinning knowledge

A number of oral or written questions may be asked relating to ventricular fibrillation, semi-automatic external defibrillators, electrocardiograms, cardiac rhythms/arrhythmias, safety precautions and care of a semi-automatic external defibrillator. Examples have been included at the end of the chapter.

practical demonstration

You may be asked to demonstrate the operation of a semi-automatic external defibrillator.

scenario

You may be required to treat one or more patients experiencing ventricular fibrillation.

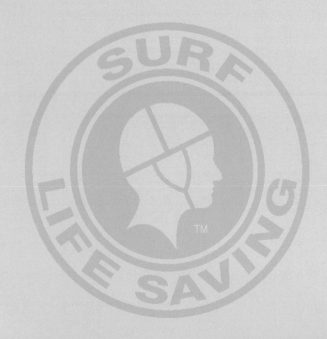

Sudden cardiac arrest is one of the leading causes of death in Australia, claiming the lives of 25 000 Australians each year.

Sudden cardiac arrest is treatable, with impressive survival statistics after immediate defibrillation. Tragically, however, this seldom occurs outside the hospital setting. Survival rates decline dramatically with each minute that passes before defibrillation.

DELAY BETWEEN NOTIFICATION AND DEFIBRILLATION	SURVIVAL RATE*
Immediate: 1–2 minutes	90%
Early: 6 minutes	45%
Early: 7 minutes	30%
Delayed: >10 minutes	<5%

*For patients with sudden cardiac arrest in witnessed ventricular fibrillation. Based on US statistics.
Source: http://www.early-defib.org/03_01_01.html
Note: Two successful defibrillation cases from SLSA occurred at 27 and 44 minutes, after continuous and effective CPR.

what is defibrillation?

Ventricular fibrillation is the rapid, irregular and unco-ordinated contraction of the heart. Defibrillation involves delivering an electric shock to revert the heart to its normal (sinus) rhythm.

A common cause of ventricular fibrillation is heart attack — a life-threatening cardiac arrhythmia where the heart ceases to function effectively and cannot pump blood to the lungs for oxygenation or pump oxygenated blood throughout the body — which will cause perma-nent damage and death if normal cardiac function is not rapidly restored. Defibrillation is the most effective method of successfully resuscitating a heart attack patient in ventricular fibrillation.

Early access to defibrillation, when combined with starting effective CPR (see Chapter 5) as early as possible, provides the best chance of survival for a patient suffering cardiac arrest. Defibrillation of the heart by first aid per-sonnel has become possible with semi-automatic external defibrillators.

what is an SAED?

The semi-automatic external defibrillator (SAED) is a portable device able to recognise shockable rhythms in a patient in cardiac arrest and able to deliver an electrical shock to revert the heart back to its normal rhythm.

chain of survival

The 'chain of survival' is a representation of basic man-agement of emergency cardiac events. The best chance a person has of surviving an out-of-hospital cardiac arrest is if the following sequence of emergency care can be initiated as quickly as possible.

+ *Early access:* this refers to the recognition of the emergency, and calling for urgent medical help as quickly as possible.
+ *Early CPR:* the manual life support system that delivers oxygen to the heart, brain and other vital organs to prevent the patient from hypoxia and deterioration. CPR must be started as soon as possible; it supports heart function until a defibrillation unit arrives.
+ *Early defibrillation:* the delivery of a precise electric shock to the heart by a defibrillator in an attempt to restore normal sinus heart rhythm. Defibrillation is, perhaps, the most important factor in influencing survival from a cardiac arrest.
+ *Early advanced life support:* the intensive care facilities and the range of life-saving drug therapies available that can be administered both in hospital and, in some cases, in the field.

Research has shown that the chances of survival from an out-of-hospital cardiac arrest can be significantly improved if each of the links in the 'chain of survival' is initiated rapidly.

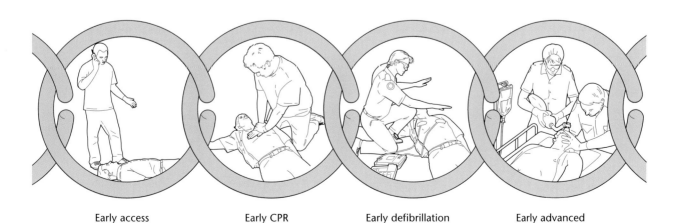

Early access   Early CPR   Early defibrillation   Early advanced life support

The chain of survival

the electro-cardiogram

The heart has two actions — a mechanical action, which is the pumping of the heart, and an electrical action, which controls the rhythmic beat of the heart.

The electrical impulse passing through the heart muscle can be mapped on a graph called an electrocardiogram (ECG). When a patient's heart is under stress or injured, changes in the electrical activity can be seen on an ECG.

The SAED measures this activity through electrodes placed on the patient's chest, and recognises life-threatening arrhythmias, such as ventricular fibrillation.

the electrical action of the heart

The electrical impulses that cause the muscle cells in the heart to contract originate in specialised pacemaker cells. The main pacemaker (the sinoatrial, or SA node) is situated in the wall of the right atrium. An electrical impulse spreads from the pacemaker through the walls of the atria, causing the muscle cells of the atria to contract and force blood into the ventricles. The electrical impulse continues down the conduction pathway to the atrioventricular (AV) node where it is momentarily slowed to allow time for the atria to contract before it spreads through the ventricles, which contract. This contraction expels blood from the heart to the lungs (from the right ventricle) or throughout the rest of the body (from the left ventricle).

In newborns and infants, the normal heart rate varies between 100 and 160 beats per minute. In children, the normal rate varies between 70 and 120 beats per minute and between 60 and 100 beats per minute in adults.

cardiac rhythm and arrhythmias

SAEDs are designed to detect life-threatening arrhythmias, such as ventricular fibrillation, and recommend defibrillation. Therefore, first aiders do not need experience in rhythm recognition — though, normal sinus rhythm and some common arrhythmias are detailed below. Some SAEDs have a display screen and manual over-ride function for use by trained health professionals.

sinus rhythm

Sinus rhythm is the normal rhythm of a healthy heart, and the SAED will *not* recommend, nor allow, a shock if normal sinus rhythm is detected.

ventricular tachycardia

Ventricular tachycardia (VT) occurs when the ventricles beat faster than the rhythm generated by the sinoatrial node. The rate will vary; however, it will always be greater than 100 beats per minute and usually no faster than 200 beats per minute. Ventricular tachycardia may be life-threatening, because it may inhibit the effective distribution of oxygenated blood throughout the body, resulting in hypoxia and organ damage. VT may progress to pulseless VT, in which case the SAED will recommend a shock.

signs
✚ Fainting
✚ Difficulty breathing or shortness of breath

symptoms
✚ Very rapid pulse or no pulse
✚ Palpitations — the patient will feel like their heart is racing
✚ Light-headedness or dizziness
✚ Angina or some type of chest pain

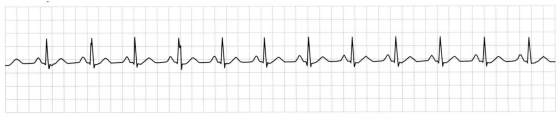

Sinus rhythm

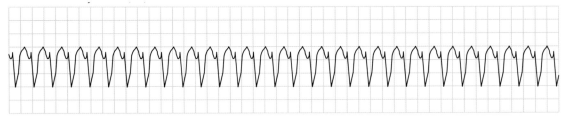

Ventricular tachycardia

treatment

In less severe cases, no treatment may be necessary and the heart will convert to normal (sinus) rhythm spontaneously. More prolonged cases of ventricular tachycardia may deteriorate into pulseless VT, which requires defibrillation. If an SAED detects this rhythm, it will recommend a shock.

ventricular fibrillation

Ventricular fibrillation (VF) is characterised by disordered electrical activity and unsynchronised, very rapid ventricular fluttering. In the absence of effective contractions, the ventricles cannot pump blood throughout the body resulting in no cardiac output and no pulse. This is a life-threatening arrhythmia that results in collapse with cardiac arrest.

signs

+ Loss of consciousness
+ No breathing, no pulse

treatment

+ DRABC.
+ Defibrillation.

asystole

There is very minimal electrical activity during ventricular asystole, but no contraction of the heart muscle and, consequently, no pulse. CPR is the only treatment. The SAED will *not* recommend a shock if this rhythm is detected.

types of SAED

monophasic

The electrical current is triggered and passes only from one pad to the other. They deliver a preset charge of 200 kJ on the first and second shocks, and then 360 kJ for the third and subsequent shocks.

biphasic

The charge goes from one pad to the other and then returns. Thus, it is possible to run them at a lower voltage, and the usual charge can be less than the monophasic models, but they are as effective.

the defibrillation process

The SAED delivers an electric shock through electrode pads applied to the patient's chest. This process stops the heart's abnormal electrical activity, restoring normal sinus rhythm and cardiac function.

Indications for the use of an SAED are:

+ the patient is unresponsive
+ the patient is not breathing
+ the patient has no pulse
+ the first aider has access to the SAED
+ the first aider is trained/certified in the use of the SAED.

When connected to a patient, the SAED will:

+ prompt specific actions
+ analyse the patient's ECG (either automatically or when activated by the operator, depending on the unit)
+ advise to shock, if an appropriate arrhythmia is detected
+ deliver a shock when activated by the operator
+ advise to recommence CPR if no shockable arrhythmia is detected.

operation of the SAED

+ Confirm that the patient needs defibrillation, i.e. that the patient is unresponsive, not breathing and has no pulse.

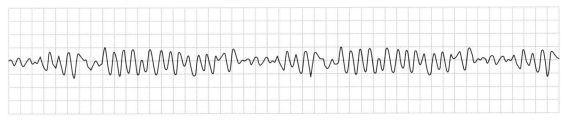

Ventricular fibrillation

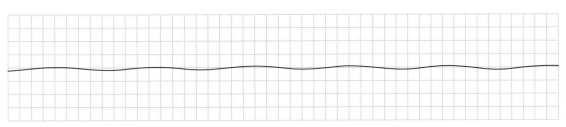

Asystole

- ✚ Always check that conditions are safe for the use of an SAED.
  - — The patient should not be lying in or on anything wet or in contact with anything metallic.
  - — Oxygen delivery units are directed away from the patient.
  - — There is nothing under the electrode pads (e.g. medication patches, pacemakers).
  - — No-one is touching the patient.
- ✚ Turn on defibrillator.
- ✚ Apply electrode pads to the patient's chest.

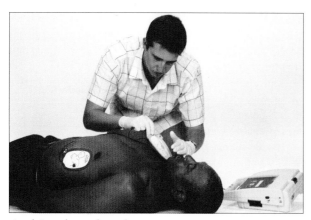

Applying electrode pads

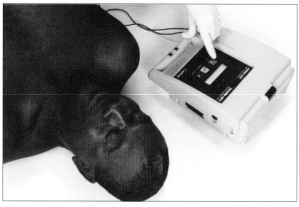

Turning the defibrillator unit on

- ✚ Respond to the unit's prompts.
- ✚ Deliver a shock in an appropriate and safe manner, as described above.
- ✚ Maintain basic life-support protocols.

 NOTE:
- • Respond to all prompts within safety constraints.
- • Make sure all personnel are clear of the patient during analysis and before delivering a shock.

effective adherence of electrode pads

The following points will help ensure effective adherence of electrode pads:

- ✚ only place electrode pads on clean, dry skin
- ✚ do not use alcohol wipes

- ✚ if the chest is hairy, remove hair with razor or shears
- ✚ apply electrode pads with a smooth rolling action to prevent air bubbles
- ✚ once applied, electrode pads should not be repositioned or removed
- ✚ do not use electrodes after their expiry date.

 NOTE:
Currently, all pads are single-use only.

positioning of electrode pads

Correct positioning of the electrode pads is essential for successful defibrillation to take place. The optimal position is usually indicated on the electrode pads or on the packaging they come in.

- ✚ Place the sternum electrode pad to the right of the sternum (breastbone) below the collarbone and above the right nipple.
- ✚ Place the apex electrode pad to the left of the sternum, with the upper edge of the pad below and to the left of the nipple.

 NOTE:
- • Do not remove electrodes after a patient's pulse has returned. Keep them in place to allow prompt action should the patient's condition deteriorate.
- • Do not place electrodes over medication patches.
- • If the patient has an implanted pacemaker, make sure that the pads are at least 10 cm away from it.

accessories

Other items that should be kept with the defibrillation unit include:

- ✚ resuscitation masks
- ✚ gloves
- ✚ razors
- ✚ shears
- ✚ gauze wipes (or similar)
- ✚ spare battery (if applicable to SAED)
- ✚ space blanket
- ✚ pen and paper
- ✚ chamois or towel.

shock delivery protocols

The normal shock delivery voltage is preset and depends if the unit is monophasic or biphasic.

Shocks are delivered in clusters of three followed by a pause for recovery, checks and resuscitation, as required.

defibrillation safety

Rescuers must operate the SAED safely. Safety considerations include, but are not limited to, the following.

+ The operator must be trained/certified in the use of the defibrillator.
+ The patient must be unresponsive, not breathing and without a pulse.
+ Remove any metallic jewellery near the electrode sites.
+ Do not place electrodes over medication patches.
+ Avoid contact between the electrodes and any metal surface.
+ Operators and bystanders must have no contact with the patient during defibrillation.
+ Do not operate the SAED in an explosive environment (e.g. where gases or fumes might be present).
+ In wet conditions (e.g. rain), wipe the chest dry before positioning electrodes. It is usually best to move the patient lying in water to a dry area.
+ If the patient has an implanted pacemaker, make sure that the pads are at least 10 cm away from it.
+ Use only equipment (e.g. electrodes, batteries) that is compatible with the unit.
+ Do not operate the unit in close proximity to mobile phones, radios, etc.
+ Do not operate the unit in an unstable environment, which may prevent it from performing a valid assessment of the ECG signal.

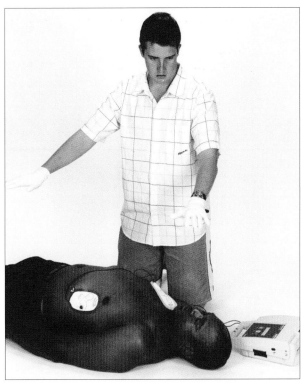

Stand clear — there must be no contact with the patient during defibrillation

SAED skills should be practised on a regular basis. This is particularly so in environments where rescuers seldom encounter patients in cardiac arrest.

SAED PROMPTS

SAED prompts may vary, depending on the make and model, but they are usually similar to those shown below.

FUNCTION	EXAMPLES
Turning on defibrillator	'Press on'
Attaching electrodes to patient	'Attach electrodes'
Initiating analysis of ECG	'Press to analyse'
Warning that charging is taking place	'Charging' — with rising audible tone
Warning not to touch patient during shock	'Stand clear' 'Do not touch the patient'
Initiating shock	'Shock advised' 'Press to shock' 'Push flashing button'
Stating that a non-shockable rhythm is present	'No shock advised' 'Check pulse' 'If no pulse, commence CPR'
Warning that ECG signal is unsatisfactory	'Check electrodes' 'Motion detected'

There may be prompts for maintenance, such as battery condition and the need for recharging or replacement.

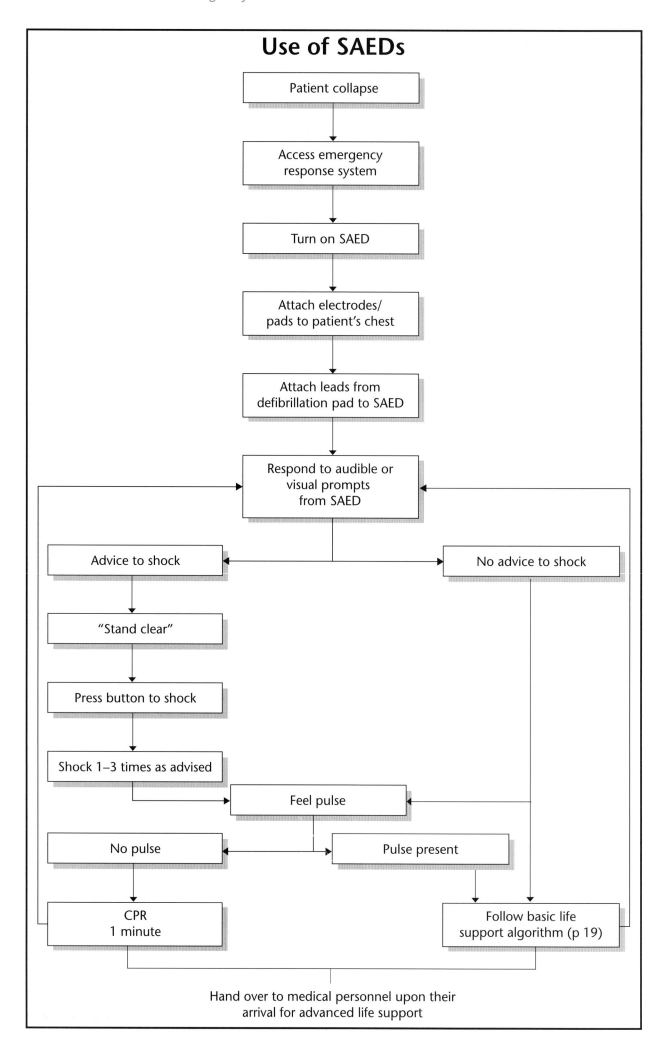

Use of SAEDs

Patient collapse

↓

Access emergency
response system

↓

Turn on SAED

↓

Attach electrodes/
pads to patient's chest

↓

Attach leads from
defibrillation pad to SAED

↓

Respond to audible or
visual prompts
from SAED

Advice to shock   ←   No advice to shock

↓

"Stand clear"

↓

Press button to shock

↓

Shock 1–3 times as advised   →   Feel pulse   ←

No pulse   ←   Pulse present

↓

CPR
1 minute

Follow basic life
support algorithm (p 19)

Hand over to medical personnel upon their
arrival for advanced life support

revision

1. What is defibrillation?

   _____

   _____

2. Complete the following sentences about the electrical action of the heart.

   The heart's main pacemaker, or .... node, are located in the wall of the right .... After

   spreading through the atria, ... impulses continue down to the .... node in the ventricles,

   causing them to ....

3. Indicate whether an SAED would recommend defibrillation or not for the following conditions:
   Y/N   Asystole.
   Y/N   Ventricular fibrillation.
   Y/N   Pulseless ventricular tachycardia.
   Y/N   Sinus rhythm.

4. List the indications for using an SAED:

   a) _____

   b) _____

   c) _____

   d) _____

   e) _____

5. Describe the correct position of the two electrode pads for defibrillation:

   a) _____

   b) _____

6. Which of the following is *not* true regarding defibrillation safety?
   a) The operator must be trained/certified in the use of the defibrillator.
   b) The patient must be unresponsive, not breathing and without a pulse.
   c) Operators and bystanders must have no contact with the patient during defibrillation.
   d) In wet conditions (e.g. rain), there is no need to wipe the chest dry before positioning electrodes.

Answers appear in Appendix 8.

pain management and administration of analgesic gases

learning outcomes

Perform pain management techniques and administration of analgesic gases during first aid and emergency care.

+ Detail the principles of pain management.
+ Demonstrate basic pain management.
+ Detail the safety considerations and procedure for administering nitrous oxide.
+ Detail the safety considerations and procedure for administering methoxyflurane.
+ Detail the documentation involved in the use of nitrous oxide and methoxyflurane.

See Appendix 7 for the safe handling of medical gases

how you may be assessed

underpinning knowledge

A number of oral or written questions may be asked relating to pain management, safety considerations when using analgesic gases, administration of analgesic gases, nitrous oxide, methoxyflurane and documenting the use of analgesic gases on patients. Examples have been included at the end of the chapter.

practical demonstration

You may be asked to demonstrate basic pain management techniques with casualties. You may be asked to demonstrate the safety considerations and administration procedure for nitrous oxide. You may be asked to demonstrate the safety considerations and administration procedure for methoxyflurane. You may be asked to demonstrate how you would document the use of analgesic gases in first aid and emergency care.

scenario

You may be required to treat one or more patients with severe pain and administer analgesic gas.

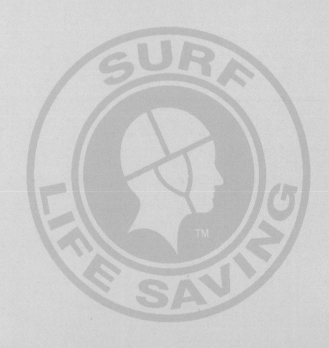

what is pain?

Pain is a sensation, ranging from mild discomfort to agony. The sensation of pain may be localised or systemic (widespread). It is caused by stimulation of pain receptors.

Nerve cells convey information from receptors (nociceptors) in the extremities and viscera (organs) of the body to the brain, where they are perceived as pain.

Pain often serves as a protective mechanism as sudden pain initiates a reflex that causes muscle contraction thereby moving the limb away from the painful stimulus, such as burns or treading on a nail.

principles of pain management

A patient suffering extreme pain can focus on little else and is often unco-operative and unwilling to help the first aider apply timely and effective treatments. A gentle, but confident and professional approach to any patient will build trust and make treatment administration easier.

Whether applying simple pain management methods such as ice, or formal pain management techniques discussed in this chapter, the principles are the same — relieve the patient's suffering, as you are unlikely to be able to stop the pain.

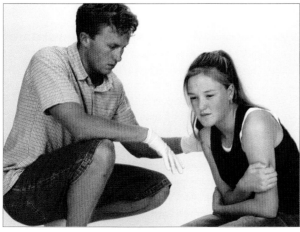

Be gentle, but confident with casualties in pain

This chapter reviews the use of the inhaled analgesics: nitrous oxide and methoxyflurane. They can relieve discomfort, but will not completely eliminate pain.

NOTE:
- Both nitrous oxide and methoxyflurane have serious side effects if over used.
- Use should only be encouraged to reach a more bearable level of pain.

basic pain management

+ Reassurance.
+ Cold packs for local skin pain (see Chapters 15, 17).
+ Heat for penetrating marine injuries (see Chapter 15).
+ Administration of nitrous oxide or methoxyflurane for severe pain.

nitrous oxide

Nitrous oxide (laughing gas) is a colourless, odourless and slightly sweet-tasting gas with analgesic properties. A mixture of 50% nitrous oxide and 50% oxygen is known as Entonox. It works quickly on the central nervous system and wears off rapidly once treatment is stopped. It also provides adequate oxygenation for conditions where oxygen therapy is indicated.

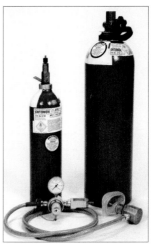

Nitrous oxide cylinders

identification

Nitrous oxide comes in a single cylinder with a blue and white quartered shoulder. It has a unique connection, so that only the nitrous oxide delivery system can be connected to a nitrous oxide cylinder.

The cylinder may display a label indicating one of the following:

+ 50% nitrous oxide
+ Entonox
+ 50% nitrous oxide / oxygen
+ Nitrous oxide:oxygen 50:50.

mode of action

On inhalation, nitrous oxide passes easily into the blood across the respiratory membrane in the lungs, in a similar way to oxygen. Nitrous oxide acts directly on the central nervous system to reduce the sensation of pain.

safety

Nitrous oxide is expelled from the patient's lungs in the same form as it is inhaled. The nitrous oxide exhaled by a patient may be absorbed and have an effect on people nearby. Care must be taken if nitrous oxide is used in confined spaces (including some first aid rooms) — use only in well-ventilated areas to avoid those treating the patient from inhaling large quantities of the drug.

Be certain that no contraindications exist before starting treatment.

contraindications

In all patients who have any contraindications, nitrous oxide will make the patient's condition worse. Nitrous oxide will diffuse into air-filled cavities faster than the air can diffuse out. Therefore, the air-filled cavity will increase in size, pressure or both.

Nitrous oxide is contraindicated in patients whom:

✚ cannot understand or comply with instructions for use as treatment is self-administered
✚ have suspected air embolus (see Chapter 9)
✚ have suspected decompression sickness (see Chapter 9)
✚ have suspected pneumothorax (see Chapter 8)
✚ have suspected bowel obstruction
✚ have a decreased level of consciousness and cannot use the apparatus themselves
✚ have impaired gas exchange (e.g. near drownings).

> **NOTE:**
> Generally, nitrous oxide is inappropriate for children under 4 years of age.

patient questioning

Be certain that none of the above contraindications exist before starting treatment. It is recommended that a checklist be kept connected to the cylinder to allow careful patient questioning before use.

dangers and difficulties in using nitrous oxide

Nitrous oxide is not flammable, but will support combustion, because of the 50% oxygen content. Care should be taken when using nitrous oxide around any naked flame.

Nitrous oxide is delivered through a demand valve, which only opens to allow gas flow when the patient inhales. The patient must inhale strongly enough to open the valve. This may not be possible in some patients, so nitrous oxide therapy will be unsuccessful. Suspect poor inhalation in patients who do not experience any pain relief.

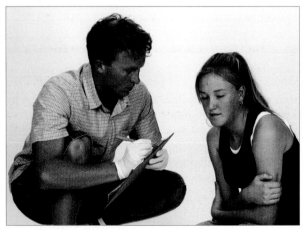

Patient questioning is important to reveal whether patients have any contraindications to treatment

If the nitrous oxide cylinder has been exposed to temperatures below 5°C, the two gases may separate (the oxygen rises to the top and the patient may be inhaling pure oxygen instead of 50% nitrous oxide and 50% oxygen). Immerse the cylinder in water no warmer than 37°C for at least 5 minutes and invert the cylinder three times to re-mix the gases.

administering nitrous oxide

The following protocol should be followed in all instances where patients are treated with nitrous oxide.
1. Reassure the patient.
2. Question the patient to ascertain that there are no contraindications to nitrous oxide treatment.
3. Explain the procedure to the patient:

> **NOTE:**
> The forms mentioned in this section will vary depending on State legislation. Specific instruction will be given in the pain management course.

   a) This is nitrous oxide, which will help relieve your pain
   b) You must hold the mask to your face while you breathe in and out
   c) The gas will only flow into the mask when you inhale. *Breathe normally*
   d) Your pain will start to ease shortly after you start inhaling, but it won't disappear completely
   e) If you feel any side effects, take the mask away from your face. The unpleasant effects will wear off fairly quickly, but your pain will also worsen.
4. Ensure the patient understands the instructions for use.
5. Invert the cylinder three times to mix the gases.
6. Upon starting treatment, record the following:
   a) In the 'Drug Register' (State specific)
      (i) date, patient's full name, date of birth
      (ii) volume meter reading
   b) On the 'Medical Response Form' (State specific)
      (i) time therapy started.
7. When a satisfactory level of pain relief is achieved, check level of consciousness by giving the patient some simple commands (e.g. lift your left arm, squeeze my hand, wiggle your toes).
8. At the end of treatment, record the following:
   a) In the 'Drug Register'
      (i) volume meter reading
   b) On the 'Medical Response Form'
      (i) time therapy stopped
      (ii) total inhalation time
      (iii) total volume inhaled.
9. As soon as nitrous oxide treatment is stopped, place the patient on oxygen therapy for at least three minutes.
10. Ensure a *completed* copy of the 'Medical Response Form' goes to hospital with the patient.

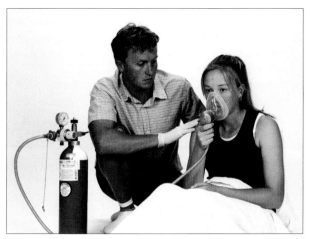

Administering nitrous oxide

Patients treated with nitrous oxide must not be allowed to leave without further medical follow-up. Generally, the injuries being treated will prevent this from happening. The patient should be transported to hospital by ambulance.

NOTE:
Only use nitrous oxide if all other pain relief options have been exhausted (i.e. reassurance, ice, heat, as appropriate).

side effects

Side effects from treatment with nitrous oxide are minor and relatively uncommon and include:

+ nausea and vomiting
+ dizziness
+ drowsiness
+ temporary loss of consciousness (rare).

When a patient stops inhaling, the nitrous oxide rapidly diffuses out of the blood into the lungs, however, oxygen therapy for 3 minutes at the completion of nitrous oxide treatment will be helpful.

methoxyflurane

Pain relief from methoxyflurane occurs more slowly than nitrous oxide (onset in 2–3 minutes) but lasts longer once treatment has stopped (4–5 minutes).

identification

Methoxyflurane is produced in a 3 mL sealed amber glass bottle. It may be labelled as one of the following:

+ methoxyflurane
+ Penthrane
+ Penthrox.

The methoxyflurane bottle and packaging will have a 'Use by' date. Never use methoxyflurane past this date. It

should be disposed of according to local authorities and replaced with fresh stock.

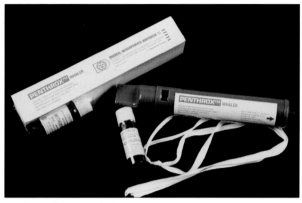

Methoxyflurane inhaler

mode of action

On inhalation, methoxyflurane passes easily into the blood across the respiratory membrane in the lungs, in a similar way to oxygen. Methoxyflurane acts directly on the central nervous system to reduce the sensation of pain.

safety

The same requirements for adequate ventilation exist as with nitrous oxide. Methoxyflurane may be harmful to the kidneys, so it is essential that methoxyflurane only be used in well-ventilated areas to avoid first aiders being exposed to the gas. It is recommended that gloves and safety glasses be worn while handling and decanting the liquid in the vial.

contraindications

Methoxyflurane is contraindicated in patients:

+ with a history of kidney disease (renal impairment or renal failure), as it may cause kidney damage
+ with a head injury or an altered state of consciousness from any cause (including alcohol). A rare complication of methoxyflurane treatment is loss of consciousness, the danger of which is multiplied in patients whom already have a depressed level of consciousness
+ with respiratory depression, as it may worsen the condition
+ with cardiovascular instability, as it may worsen circulatory depression.

patient questioning
Be certain that none of the above contraindications exist before starting treatment. All patients considered for treatment with methoxyflurane must be asked if they have a history of kidney disease.

dangers and difficulties in using methoxyflurane
While administering methoxyflurane, be vigilant for signs of respiratory or circulatory depression and loss of consciousness.

Methoxyflurane is a highly volatile liquid, as it may ignite under relatively normal conditions. The flashpoint (lowest temperature for the vapour above a liquid to be ignited in air) of methoxyflurane is 62.8°C in air and 32.8°C when mixed with oxygen. It is important that the methoxyflurane bottle is not left in direct sunlight. Methoxyflurane ignites easily and extra care should be taken when using supplemental oxygen therapy in the presence of naked flames or in other flammable situations.

administering methoxyflurane

Methoxyflurane is self-administered by the patient through an inhaler, which is disposable and for single use only. The inhaler has an oxygen therapy port for supplemental oxygen if required. As with nitrous oxide, self-administration ensures that if the patient loses consciousness the inhaler will fall away from the face and the patient will inhale room air.

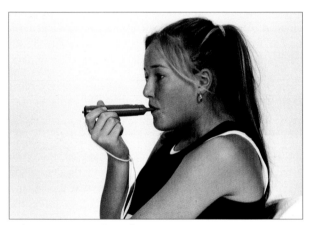

Administering methoxyflurane

1. Reassure the patient.
2. Ascertain that there are no contraindications to methoxyflurane treatment.
3. Explain the procedure to the patient:
   a) This is methoxyflurane, which will help relieve your pain
   b) You must take the inhaler in your mouth while you breathe in
   c) The gas will only be inhaled when you breathe in
   d) Continue inhaling until the pain starts to dull. Aim for relief of discomfort rather than complete abolition of pain
   e) If you feel any side effects, remove the inhaler. The unpleasant effects will wear off, but your pain will also worsen.
4. Ensure the patient understands the instructions for use.
5. Hold the inhaler vertically with the mouthpiece down. Open the vial and pour the full 3 mL into the base cap. Shake gently and wipe the mouthpiece.
6. If possible, connect the oxygen therapy tube to the nipple on the inhaler and administer the gas with oxygen therapy running.

7. After the patient has taken 8–10 breaths, they can be instructed to place their finger over the diluter hole to increase the concentration of methoxyflurane they are inhaling.
8. Instruct the patient to inhale the methoxyflurane intermittently but sufficiently to provide adequate pain relief.
9. Fasten the strap of the inhaler to the patient's wrist.
10. Upon starting treatment, record the following:
    a) In the 'Drug Register'
       (i) date, patient's full name, date of birth
       (ii) time therapy started.
    b) On the 'Medical Response Form'
       (i) time therapy started.
11. When a satisfactory level of pain relief is achieved, check level of consciousness by giving the patient some simple commands (e.g. lift your left arm, squeeze my hand, wiggle your toes). Continually assess the patient's level of consciousness as long as they are inhaling methoxyflurane.
12. At the end of treatment, record the following:
    a) In the 'Drug Register'
       (i) time therapy stopped
    b) On the 'Medical Response Form'
       (i) time therapy stopped.
       (ii) total inhalation time.
13. If the first dose of methoxyflurane runs out, a second vial can be used. The total dose administered must not exceed 6 mL (i.e. 2 vials max).
14. As soon as methoxyflurane treatment is stopped, place the patient on oxygen therapy for at least 3 minutes.
15. Ensure a *completed* copy of the 'Medical Response Form' goes to hospital with the patient.

Patients treated with methoxyflurane must not be allowed to leave without further medical follow-up. The patient should be transported to hospital by ambulance.

side effects

+ Nausea
+ Vomiting
+ Headache
+ Skin irritation

Serious side effects are:

+ profound respiratory and circulatory depression
+ loss of consciousness
+ severe kidney disease.

documentation

Specific legislation regarding the storage, use of and documentation for nitrous oxide and methoxyflurane will vary from State to State. Specific legislation will be discussed during your pain management course.

revision

1. Complete the following sentence about the principles of pain management.

   Whether applying .... methods such as ice, or .... pain management techniques,

   the .... are the same — relieve the patient's ...., as you are unlikely to be able to stop the

   ....

2. List the types of basic pain management:

   a) _____

   b) _____

   c) _____

   d) _____

   e) _____

3. What is Entonox?

   _____

   _____

4. List five contraindications for nitrous oxide therapy:

   a) _____

   b) _____

   c) _____

   d) _____

   e) _____

5. What are the most common side effects of nitrous oxide therapy?

   a) _____   b) _____

   c) _____   d) _____

6. List the contraindications for methoxyflurane therapy:

   a) _____

   b) _____

   c) _____

   d) _____

7. What are the side effects of methoxyflurane therapy?

   a) _____   b) _____

   c) _____   d) _____

8. What are the potential serious side effects of methoxyflurane therapy?

   a) _____

   b) _____

   c) _____

Answers appear in Appendix 8.

appendices

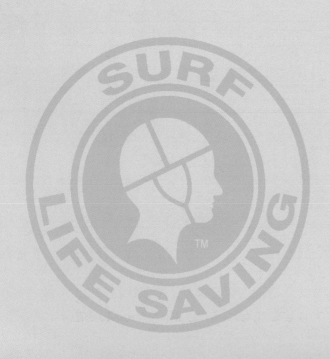

appendix one:
first aid documentation form

SURF LIFE SAVING AUSTRALIA LTD.

Incident Report Log

Name of Club or Service: _____

State: _____

Details of Incident

Date: ____/____/_____ Time: _____ am / pm

Location of Incident: _____

Name of Victim _____

Age: _____ DOB: ____/____/_____ M / F

Address if known _____

Venue Conditions at Time of incident: (if relevant)

Wind conditions: ❑ Calm ❑ Slight ❑ Moderate
Weather conditions: ❑ Fine ❑ Overcast ❑ Rain
Sea conditions: ❑ Small ❑ Medium ❑ Large
Water surface: ❑ No chop ❑ Avg chop ❑ Large chop
Wave type: ❑ Surging ❑ Spilling ❑ Plunging

Please fill in the below relating to the victim

Type of Incident: (may cross more than one)
❑ [1]Major First Aid ❑ [2]Minor FA*
❑ [3]Major Rescue ❑ [4]S & R
❑ [5]Member Injury ❑ [6]Employee Injury
❑ [7]Carnival Incident ❑ [8]Complaint
❑ [9]Drowning ❑ [10]Near Drowning
❑ [11]Other_____

Victim is:
❑ [1]Public ❑ [2]SLS Club Member
❑ [3]Employee ❑ [4]Other _____

Postcode of usual residence (victim)
_____ or ❑ [1]Unknown
❑ [2]Overseas ❑ [3]No fixed address

Type of activity at time of incident:
❑ [1]Swimming/wading ❑ [2]Body board
❑ [3]Walking playing near water
❑ [4]Riding other craft
❑ [5]Rock Fishing ❑ [6]Other fishing
❑ [7]Using a motorised water craft (Rec)
❑ [8]Water skiing
❑ [9]SCUBA/skin diving
❑ [10]Wind/kite surfing ❑ [11]Sailing
❑ [12]Rock walking
❑ [13]Suspected suicide

❑ [14]Patrolling in - ❑ [15]IRB, ❑ [16]PWC
❑ [17]Beach, ❑ [18]4WD ❑ [19]JRB/ORB
❑ [20]Attempting a rescue
❑ [21]Training for (please be very specific_____
❑ [22]Carnival Official doing _____
❑ [23]Competition in _____
❑ [24]Driver ❑ [25]Crew ❑ [26]Patient
❑ [27]Surf Boat Crew Position: _____
❑ [28]Administrative ❑ [29]Fundraising
❑ [30]Water safety
❑ [31]Junior activities
❑ [32]Other club activity_____
❑ [33]Other _____

Experience in activity
❑ [1]3 years + ❑ [2]1-3 Years
❑ [3]1 year ❑ [4]No experience

Other Contributing Factors:
❑ [1]Negotiating the break
❑ [2]Returning to shore
❑ [3]Dumped ❑ [4]Shore break
❑ [5]Lost control of own craft
❑ [6]Other person lost control of craft
❑ [7]Freak wave ❑ [8]Sand bank
❑ [9]Pot hole ❑ [12]Slippery rocks
❑ [10]Suspected Alcohol ❑ [11]Suspect Drugs
❑ [13]Rip type _____
❑ [14]Slip/ trip/ fall ❑ [16]Assault
❑ [15]Collision with _____
❑ [17]Mechanical Malfunction_____
❑ [18]Other _____

Description of Incident (please use back if needed)_____
_____
_____
_____
_____

Nature of Injury
❑ [1]Marine Sting, type _____
❑ [2]Abrasion / graze ❑ [3]Blisters
❑ [4]Open wound /laceration / cut
❑ [5]Bruise / contusion
❑ [6]Inflammation / swelling
❑ [7]Fracture (including suspected)
❑ [8]Dislocation/subluxation
❑ [9]Sprain ❑ [10]Strain
❑ [11]Overuse injury ❑ [12]Concussion
❑ [13]Cardiac problem
❑ [14]Respiratory problem
❑ [15]Loss of consciousness
❑ [16]Heat stroke / Heat exhaustion
❑ [17]Hypothermia ❑ [18]Sunburn
❑ [19]Suspected spinal
❑ [20]Deceased
❑ [21]Other_____

Body region injured: (Please Circle)

Description _____

Initial treatment:
❑ [1]None given – not required
❑ [2]None given – patient refused
❑ [3]None given – referred elsewhere
❑ [4]RICE ❑ [4]ICE
❑ [5]Cleaned
❑ [6]Dressed (Incl. Bandage)
❑ [7]Sling / Splint
❑ [8]Spinal collar
❑ [9]Massage / Stretching
❑ [10]Strapping/Taping only
❑ [11]Stitches
❑ [12]Medication
❑ [13]Prescription written

Resuscitation
(Please fill in other side of form)
❑ [14]EAR ❑ [15]CPR
❑ [16]Oxygen therapy
❑ [17]Oxygen airbag
❑ [18]Defibrillation (Defib)
❑ [19]Other_____

Mechanism of Incident (what went wrong)_____
_____
_____
_____

Location of incident?
❑ [1]In water ❑ [2]On Beach
❑ [3]On rocks ❑ [4]Other _____
and...
❑ [1]In flags
❑ [2]Outside but near flags
❑ [3]<1km from patrolled area
❑ [4]1 to 5 km from patrolled area
❑ [5]> 5 km from patrolled area

Who first sighted the rescue/ incident?
e.g. public_____

Who conducted the rescue/ incident?
e.g. lifesaver _____

Main Language Spoken:
_____Or ❑ English
❑ Non English speaking ❑ Don't know

Referral:
❑ [1]No referral
❑ [2]Medical Practitioner
❑ [3]Physiotherapist
❑ [4]Ambulance transport to _____
❑ [5]Hospital ❑ [6]Xray
❑ [7]Peer Counselling
❑ [8]Professional Counselling

Other Services:
❑ [1]Fire/ Rescue ❑ [2]Police
❑ [3]JRB/ ORB ❑ [4]Helicopter
❑ [5]Investigation required
❑ [6]Worker Compensation required (fill in State form requirements)
❑ [7]Other_____

Treating Person:
❑ [1]Medical Practitioner ❑ [2]Nurse
❑ [3]Ambulance ❑ [4]Physiotherapist
❑ [5]Chiropractor ❑ [6]First Aid Officer
❑ [7]Lifesaving ❑ [8]Lifeguard
❑ [9]Other_____

Person Completing from:
Name_____
Position: _____
Phone: _____
Email: _____
Signature:

Forward copy to appropriate club or service officer

appendix two:
first aid kit

Depending on State regulations, the contents of a first aid kit may include the items illustrated below.

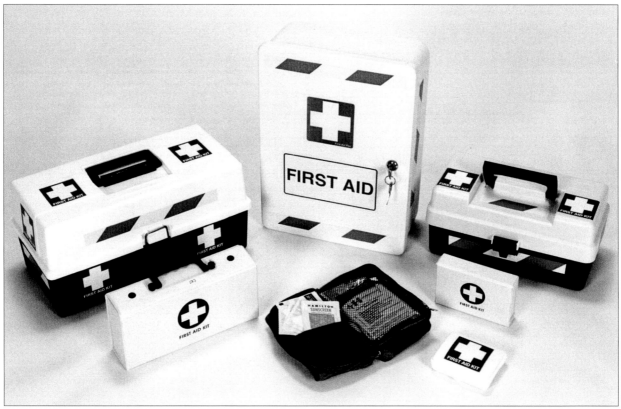

A typical first aid kit

minimum suggested contents

✚ SLSA first aid and emergency care manual.
✚ The following instruments:
  — 1 pair bandage scissors
  — 1 pair splinter forceps
  — 12 safety pins (assorted sizes).
✚ The following dressings (or equivalent sizes):
  — 25 sterile bandages (25 mm × 75 mm), individually wrapped
  — 25 sterile gauze squares (101 mm × 101 mm), individually wrapped
  — 4 rolls sterile gauze bandage (50 mm × 9 mm), individually wrapped
  — 4 rolls sterile gauze bandages (101 mm × 9 mm), individually wrapped
  — 6 triangular bandages
  — 4 sterile bandage compresses (101 mm × 101 mm), individually wrapped
  — 1 roll adhesive tape (25 mm × 9 mm).
✚ Antiseptics:
  — 25 alcohol swabs, individually wrapped.

in addition

✚ Gloves.
✚ Disposable emergency blanket.
✚ Instant cold pack.
✚ Instant hot pack.
✚ CPR pocket mask with O$_2$ inlet.

appendix three: anatomical terms of reference and comparison

The following tables explain the anatomical terms of relationship and comparison. This terminology refers to the body in what is described as the anatomical position — standing erect, looking forward with the palms of the hand and toes facing forward.

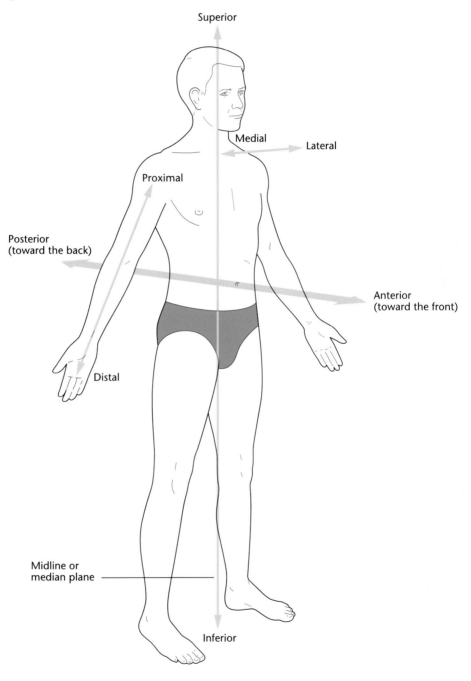

Superior

Medial — Lateral

Proximal

Posterior (toward the back)

Anterior (toward the front)

Distal

Midline or median plane

Inferior

TERMS OF RELATIONSHIP	
Anterior	Nearer to the front of the body
Posterior	Nearer to the back of the body
Superior	Nearer to the top of the head
Inferior	Nearer to the soles of the feet
Medial	Nearer to the midline of the body
Lateral	Away from the midline of the body

TERMS OF COMPARISON	
Proximal	Nearer to the body
Distal	Farther from the body
Superficial	Near to the surface or on the surface
Deep	Farther from the surface
Internal (inner)	Towards the interior
External (outer)	Towards the exterior
Ipsilateral	On the same side of the body
Contralateral	On the opposite side of the body

appendix four: patient questioning

+ What is your name?
+ I'm trained in first aid, will you let me help you?
+ What happened?
+ Are you in any pain? Where?
+ Can you take a deep breath? (to reveal chest injuries)
+ Do you have any medical conditions?
+ Are you taking any medication?
+ Are you allergic to anything?
+ When did you last have something to eat or drink?

Appropriate questions can be remembered by the acronym SAMPLE:

+ **S** signs and symptoms
+ **A** allergies
+ **M** medication
+ **P** previous medical history
+ **L** last oral intake
+ **E** event.

It is important to reassure patients as they are often scared, especially children. Children may not be able to answer these questions properly, so it may be necessary to question a parent or guardian. If the patient is unconscious or has an altered level of consciousness, there may be companions or bystanders who may have witnessed the incident who can be questioned. You can make the patient feel less anxious by remaining calm, speaking clearly and simply, reassuring the patient and referring to them by name.

If the patient is in pain, the PQRST pain assessment tool may be used:

+ **P** provocation or relief. Does anything provoke the pain (e.g. breathing, walking) or does anything make it better (e.g. resting, certain position)
+ **Q** quality of the pain. Have the patient try to identify the quality of the pain (e.g. sharp, stabbing, heavy, crushing, dull, cramping)
+ **R** radiation/region. Where is the pain and does it radiate to other parts of the body?
+ **S** severity. Have the patient rate the pain on a scale from 1 to 10, where 1 is very little pain and 10 is the most severe pain ever experienced.
+ **T** time of onset. When did the pain start and how long has the patient been in pain?

See Chapters 15 and 25 on pain management principles and approaches.

appendix five:
Glasgow coma scale

THE GLASGOW COMA SCALE		SCORE
EYE OPENING		
Spontaneous	❏	4
To speech	❏	3
To pain	❏	2
None	❏	1
BEST VERBAL RESPONSE		
Oriented conversation	❏	5
Confused conversation	❏	4
Inappropriate words	❏	3
Incomprehensible sounds	❏	2
None	❏	1
BEST MOTOR RESPONSE		
Obeys commands	❏	6
Localises pain	❏	5
Withdrawal from pain	❏	4
Abnormal flexion	❏	3
Abnormal extension	❏	2
None	❏	1

The Glasgow coma scale (GCS) is divided into three sections:

1. eye opening

✚ Observe the patient. If their eyes are open, record a score in the 'Spontaneous' box.
✚ If the patient responds to their name being called, record a score in the 'To speech' box.
✚ If the patient fails to respond to voice but opens their eyes to pressure/painful stimuli, record a score in the 'To pain' box.
✚ If the patient's eyes are closed because of swelling (head trauma or anaphylaxis), record a C (for closed) in the 'None' box. If only one eye is swollen or the patient has a glass eye, record the observations of the healthy eye.
✚ If the patient's eyes do not open with any sort of stimulus, record a score in the 'None' box.

2. best verbal response

✚ If the patient can correctly answer simple, relevant questions (such as time and place) either verbally, through an interpreter or in writing, record a score in the 'Orientated conversation' box.

✚ If the patient gives an incorrect answer to a simple question, record a score in the 'Confused conversation' box.
✚ If the patient's reply is not related to the question, but their speech is still comprehensible, record a score in the 'Inappropriate words' box.
✚ If the patient's reply is totally incoherent (e.g. mumbling), record a score in the 'Incomprehensible sounds' box.
✚ If the patient makes no reply at all to either verbal questions or physical stimuli, record a score in the 'None' box.

3. best motor response

✚ If the patient is awake and alert and responds to simple requests/commands, record a score in the 'Obeys commands' box.
✚ If the patient appears unresponsive, squeeze their shoulder and shout at them. Use a sternal rub to see if the patient can localise pain by moving their hand to the source of the stimulus in an attempt to remove it. Only a small amount of pressure is required. Then record a score in the 'Localises pain' box.
✚ If the patient does not readily respond by localising, then apply nail bed pressure to determine if the patient withdraws their hand. If the patient attempts to pull away from the stimuli, record a score in the 'Withdrawal from pain' box.
✚ If the patient is paralysed down one side (hemiplegic), record either L or R, depending on which limbs respond, in the 'Obeys commands', 'Localises pain' or 'Withdrawal from pain' boxes, along with a score next to it.
✚ If the patient responds to painful/pressure stimuli to the arm by rotating it into an abnormal flexion position (also known as *decorticate posture*), record a score in the 'Abnormal flexion' box.
✚ If the patient responds to painful stimuli to the arm by rotating it medially and extending the forearm (also known as *decerebrate posture*), record a score in the 'Abnormal extension' box.
✚ Where the patient is already decorticate or decerebrate on initial assessment and their position doesn't change with stimuli, record a score in the 'None' box.
✚ Where the patient is unresponsive to stimuli and remains flaccid, record a score in the 'None' box.

A score between 3 and 15 will be recorded. Some key GCS landmarks are as follows:

GCS 15 = Conscious, orientated to time and place.

GCS 9+ = Altered conscious state, unlikely to accept an airway but may be inadequately ventilated.

GCS 5 = Altered conscious state, loss of gag reflex.

GCS 3 = Unconscious, unresponsive to pain, absent muscle tone (flaccid).

A GCS of ≥13 6 hours after injury correlates with a mild brain injury, 9 to 12 is a moderate injury and 8 or less is a severe brain injury.

appendix six:
the APGAR score

The APGAR score

An APGAR score indicates a baby's condition and response to any resuscitation attempts. Scores are taken at 1 and 5 minutes after delivery. Scores of 0, 1 or 2 are assigned on the following criteria.

Appearance (colour)
0: Baby is uniformly blue or pale
1: Pink body with blue hands or feet
2: Completely pink all over

Pulse (heart rate)
0: No pulse
1: < 100 beats per minute
2: > 100 beats per minute

Grimace (reflex irritability)
0: No response to stimulation or airways being suctioned
1: Grimace during stimulation or suctioning
2: Grimace, pulls away, coughs or sneezes during stimulation or suctioning

Activity
0: No movement, appears limp and floppy
1: Some flexing (bending) of limbs
2: Active spontaneous motion

Respiration:
0: Not breathing
1: Slow irregular breathing, weak crying, whimpering or grunting
2: Normal respiratory rate, good, strong crying

appendix seven: safe handling of medical gases

10 steps to safe handling of medical gases

1. Store in well-ventilated areas.
2. Secure upright with restraint.
3. Keep full and empty cylinders separate.
4. Keep free of sources of ignition.
5. Wear safety shoes and gloves.
6. Always move cylinders with an appropriate trolley.
7. Never knock violently or allow to fall.
8. Keep free of oil and grease.
9. Read labels before use.
10. Do not force valves when opening or closing.

cylinder identification

+ Medical gas cylinders are identified by the information on the cylinder label, cylinder valve outlet, gas code and cylinder colour.
+ Cylinder sizes are identified by a letter code (G, E, D, C) shown on the label.
+ The nominal content is shown in litres.

+ For all cylinders containing liquid gases (e.g. carbon dioxide, nitrous oxide), the tare or empty weight of the cylinder is stamped on the aluminium ring located under the valve.

material safety data sheets

In addition to the information on the cylinder labels, Material Safety Data sheets provide further information on each of the different medical gases.

personal protection

When moving cylinders, it is good practice to wear safety shoes and gloves. All personnel handling gas cylinders should have knowledge of the properties of the gas and the precautions to be taken when handling the gas.

storing cylinders

Medical gas cylinders should be kept in a purpose-designed area that preferably allows cylinders to be kept dry and in a clean condition. When designing the cylinder storage area, a risk assessment should be carried out to ensure that the chosen location is as safe as is practicable and that manual handling issues are resolved at the planning stage in line with dangerous goods legislation and AS4332.

appendix eight: answers to revision questions

chapter one: introduction to first aid

1. c.
2. All accidents and incidents that occur in the workplace, as well as accidents that occur on work premises outside working hours.
3. Commonwealth and State occupational/workplace health and safety legislation places a duty on employers to provide <u>information</u>, instruction, <u>training</u> and supervision to employees to enable them to perform their work in a safe manner without risk to <u>health</u>.
4. Any five of the following: obstructions, spills and slippery surfaces, faulty maintenance, environmental causes, incorrect storage, incorrect use of equipment, lifting and carrying, infection.
5. a) Actual consent.
   b) Implied consent.
6. a) Immunisation.
   b) Barrier methods.
   c) Hygiene.
7. a) Proving that the first aider owed a duty of care to the injured person and the standard of care required by that duty was breached.
   b) Proving that damage was caused by the breach of the duty of care.
   c) Proving that the event was reasonably foreseeable.
8. Incidents should be documented to protect the injured person, the first aider and, if in the workplace, the employer in the event of legal action. Documentation can be used to support insurance, compensation or workers compensation claims. Continuing documentation of injuries allows for the collection of data on hazards within a workplace and helps first aiders provide the best possible care for the types of injuries likely to be sustained.

chapter two: anatomy and physiology

1. Descriptive terminology is necessary to describe the position and relationship of different structures to each other without ambiguity.
2. a) Sprains.
   b) Strains.
   c) Fractures.
   d) Dislocations.
3. The upper respiratory tract includes the nostrils, nasal cavity, mouth, pharynx (throat) and larynx (voice box).
4. The lower respiratory tract consists of the trachea, bronchi and alveoli (terminal air sacs).
5. The heart has four chambers, two <u>atria</u>, which <u>receive</u> blood to pump to the ventricles, and two ventricles, one that pumps blood to the <u>lungs</u> (right), and another that pumps blood to the body (<u>left</u>).
6. a) The carotid artery in the neck.
   b) The brachial artery at the elbow (mainly felt in infants).
   c) The radial artery at the wrist.
   d) The femoral artery in the groin.
7. a) Maintain tissue fluid balance.
   b) Absorb fats and other substances from the digestive system.
   c) Assist immunity (the body's defence system).
8. a) The cerebral hemispheres are responsible for movement, senses, memory and higher cognitive function.
   b) The cerebellum is involved in motor control, muscle co-ordination and muscle tone.
   c) The brainstem is responsible for basic life-support functions, including heartbeat and respiration.

9. a) Dermis.
   b) Epidermis.
   c) Hypodermis.
10. d.

chapter three: first aid management

1. A sign is something that can be seen (objective evidence).
2. A symptom is something a person can describe (subjective evidence).
3. a) Early access.
   b) Early cardiopulmonary resuscitation.
   c) Early defibrillation.
   d) Early advanced life support.
4. d.
5. c.
6. d.
7. <u>2</u> Shoulders and front of chest, abdomen and pelvis including ribs.
   <u>5</u> Back.
   <u>3</u> Front and back of upper limbs.
   <u>1</u> Neck, up over head and down across face.
   <u>4</u> Front and back of lower limbs.
8. a) The events leading up to the incident.
   b) What happened to the patient.
   c) The patient's vital signs and times assessed.
   d) Any injuries the patient has sustained.
   e) All treatment provided by the first aider.

chapter four: expired air resuscitation (EAR)

1. During <u>inspiration</u> (inhalation), oxygen diffuses into the <u>capillaries</u> surrounding the alveoli in the lungs and <u>carbon dioxide</u> diffuses into the alveoli. Air from the <u>lungs</u> is then expelled during expiration (<u>exhalation</u>).
2. Look: look at the chest and upper abdomen, checking for movement to indicate breathing; Listen: listen for sounds of air entering and leaving the lungs, with your ear about 5 cm from the patient's nose and mouth; Feel: with your cheek over the patient's mouth and nose, feel for any movement of air. Also feel for movement of the upper abdomen or lower chest.
3. Encourage the patient to cough and observe their progress; reassure the patient; proceed with percussion and lateral chest thrusts, as appropriate for the person's age, if coughing does not remove the obstruction.
4. b.
5. A person who regurgitates or vomits while lying face up is very likely to inhale some of the stomach contents into the lungs, which may lead to serious lung damage and infection. They are also at risk of choking.
6. Any five of the following: the head is relatively large, the neck is relatively short, the tongue is large, the trachea (windpipe) is soft and easily compressed, the adenoids may be large.

chapter five: cardiopulmonary resuscitation (CPR)

1. a.
2. a) Unconsciousness.
   b) Absence of breathing.
   c) Absence of movement.
   d) Absence of the carotid pulse.
   e) Skin colour that is pale or cyanosed (blue).
3. c.
4. b.
5. d.
6. CPR is more difficult to perform on women who are in the late stages of pregnancy because the expanding uterus places upward pressure on the diaphragm making EAR and chest expansion more difficult. Also, compression may cause regurgitation and aspiration of the stomach contents.

7. In the late stages of pregnancy, the uterus may compress the major abdominal veins, impeding the return of deoxygenated blood to the heart, if the woman is placed flat on her back.
8. a) Continuation poses a danger to the first aider.
   b) Someone takes over.
   c) You cannot physically continue.
   d) The patient is pronounced dead (this can only be done, legally, by a medical doctor).
   e) Defibrillation starts.
9. d.

chapter six: bleeding

1. Remember to apply <u>direct</u> pressure, raise the <u>wound</u> if possible, rest and <u>reassure</u> the patient and <u>send</u> for medical help.
2. b.
3. c.
4. a) Nausea.
   b) Abdominal pain.
   c) Feeling faint.
5. a) A cut has penetrated the skull.
   b) An object is embedded in the skull.
   c) There is evidence of skull fracture, such as sunken, deformed areas, visible bone fragments or the brain is exposed.
6. Sit the patient with their head bent <u>forward</u>. Squeeze the <u>soft</u> part of the nostrils just below the <u>bone</u> between the thumb and forefinger for up to <u>10</u> minutes.

chapter seven: shock

1. b.
2. Hypovolaemic shock is caused by inadequate blood volume (loss of one fifth or more of the normal blood volume), due to blood loss or excessive loss of body fluids.
3. Septic shock is caused by systemic infection, leading to dilation of blood vessels and, therefore, reduced blood pressure and blood flow to the tissues.
4. a) Faintness or dizziness.
   b) Trembling or weakness in the arms and legs.
   c) Nausea.
   d) Restlessness, anxiety.
5. Lay the person on their back in a horizontal position with their legs raised. Do not elevate the head.
6. Do not raise the legs.

chapter eight: respiratory emergencies

1. b.
2. Drowning is death by <u>suffocation</u> from immersion in <u>water</u> or other <u>fluid</u>.
3. a) Strangled voice sound.
   b) Inspiratory and expiratory stridor.
   c) Extreme difficulty breathing with the use of accessory breathing muscles.
   d) Respiratory failure in severe cases.
4. Remain calm and reassure the patient. Encourage them to take slow, deep breaths. It may be useful to have the person breathe through one nostril only (closing the mouth), or breathe through pursed lips. This will reduce oxygen intake and allow carbon dioxide levels to normalise. Continue breath coaching the patient until symptoms return to normal. Seek urgent medical assistance, if initial treatment is unsuccessful.
5. Asthma is a reversible, inflammatory disease of the small airways.
6. d.
7. Pneumothorax is the build-up of <u>air</u> in the space between the two membrane layers around the <u>lungs</u>.
8. a) Respiratory distress.
   b) Shallow rapid respirations.
   c) Increased heart rate.

9. During paradoxical respirations, the floating segment of rib will move in the opposite direction to the rest of the ribs. Hence, when the patient breathes in and their chest moves out, the flail or floating segment moves inwards.

chapter nine: cardiovascular emergencies

1. a) Family history (heredity).
   b) Being male.
   c) Increasing age.
2. a) Atherosclerosis is called coronary heart disease when it affects the vessels around the heart.
   b) Atherosclerosis is called cerebrovascular disease when it affects the vessels in the brain.
   c) Atherosclerosis is called peripheral vascular disease when it affects the vessels in the limbs.
3. a) Pulse.
   b) State of consciousness.
   c) Skin colour.
   d) Skin temperature.
4. Pain, <u>tightness</u> or heaviness in the centre of the <u>chest</u>, which may radiate down either <u>arm</u>, although commonly the left, and into the <u>neck</u>, back or jaw.
5. Cardiac arrest is defined as the absence of breathing and a pulse.
6. a.
7. a) Facial droop.
   b) Motor weakness.
   c) Speech.
8. Any five of the following: acute shortness of breath, noisy gurgling breathing, rapid or irregular pulse, cough, grey, blue (cyanosed) or pale and clammy skin, swelling of the legs and/or ankles (oedema), decreased urine output.
9. a) Pain and tenderness in one limb.
   b) Red limb that is warm to the touch.
   c) Sudden-onset oedema (swelling) of the limb.
10. a) Air embolism is more likely to be seen by the first aider.
    b) Decompression illness usually presents after the dive and is less likely for the first aider to need to treat.

chapter ten: conditions affecting level of consciousness

1. Consciousness ranges from full <u>awareness</u>/responsiveness and <u>orientation</u> in time and place to <u>unconsciousness</u>, being unaware of one's surroundings and unresponsive to <u>stimulation</u>.
2. Any five of the following: traumatic injury to the head, drugs, poisons or toxic fumes, metabolic disorders, neurological disorders, lack of oxygen to the brain, swelling or bleeding within the brain, envenomation.
3. d.
4. b.
5. Febrile convulsions occur in children under the age of 5 years, in association with any illness that produces a rapid rise in body temperature. They do not indicate that the child has epilepsy.
6. Hypoglycaemia and hyperglycaemia. Hypoglycaemia has a rapid onset and needs urgent attention and, as such, is more likely to be seen by a first aider. In contrast, hyperglycaemia develops more slowly, and is less likely to be seen by a first aider.
7. Any five of the following: pallor, excessive sweating, rapid pulse, seizures, altered state of consciousness or loss of consciousness, the person may be wearing a MedicAlert tag.
8. Treatment includes assisting the person take some fast-acting sugar (e.g. sugar, juice, glucose gel, soft drinks) to elevate blood glucose level. On recovery, the person should eat some high-carbohydrate food and drink some juice.
9. Hyperglycaemia is more difficult to diagnose than hypoglycaemia and an ambulance should be called to assist. Ambulance personnel can administer insulin injections to lower blood sugar levels. Never give the conscious person any sugary substances to eat or drink, as this will increase their blood sugar levels further.

10. a) Concussion.
    b) Contusion.
    c) Compression.
    d) Penetrating injury.

chapter eleven: wounds

1. a) Minor wounds include cuts and abrasions and minor lacerations and avulsions.
   b) Puncture wounds include wounds caused by needles and nails.
   c) Major wounds include major bleeds and penetrating injuries.
2. It is beneficial to clean minor wounds (less than 2 cm in length and not deep enough to expose the underlying fat) and puncture wounds to avoid infection and minimise scarring from embedded particles. Never wash major wounds, especially after they have stopped bleeding.
3. After treating the person, locate the amputated part and place it in a clean, dry plastic bag, and seal it. Place this sealed bag on a bed of ice and water in a suitable container. Ensure that the amputated part is sent to hospital with the patient.
4. By sealing an air-tight dressing on three sides to allow air to exit, but not enter.
5. If the person is old enough to suck on the tooth to clean it allow them to do so. If the person is too young or unconscious, rinse the tooth in milk, *not* water. If the person is old enough to store the tooth in their mouth to keep it moist, place it between their gum and cheek. If the person is too young or unconscious, wrap the tooth in plastic wrap. Do not let the person rinse their mouth out.
6. Any of the following: pain in or behind the eye, spasm of the eyelids, continuous flow of tears from the eye, red eye, bleeding around the eye in severe cases, impaired or altered vision.
7. a) Deafness or significantly impaired hearing.
   b) Fluid drainage from the ear.
   c) Elevated temperature, if it occurs in conjunction with an ear infection.

chapter twelve: dressings and bandages

1. a) To soak up blood and other fluid.
   b) To assist the body in forming a clot around the wound.
   c) To protect wounds from infection.
2. a) To control bleeding.
   b) To prevent swelling.
   c) To restrict movement.
   d) To provide support.
   e) To protect and keep a wound clean.
3. d.

chapter thirteen: splints and slings

1. a) To immobilise a wounded body part.
   b) To minimise pain.
   c) To minimise movement.
   d) Restrict further injury.
2. a) Soft splints: bandages, towels, blankets, pillows.
   b) Rigid splints: board, metal strips, sticks, magazines, rolled newspaper.
   c) Body splints: adjacent fingers, chest, uninjured leg.
3. a) The arm sling.
   b) The collar-and-cuff sling.
   c) The elevation sling.

chapter fourteen: poisoning

1. a) Acute poisoning.
   b) Venomous bites and stings.
   c) Drug interactions.
2. Any five of the following: perfume, aftershave, hair dye, nail polish and nail polish remover, mouthwash, toothpaste, deodorant, cosmetics.

3. a) Swallowing or ingesting poisons.
   b) Breathing or inhaling poisons.
   c) Absorbing poisons.
   d) Injecting poisons.
4. a.
5. Any five of the following: altered level of consciousness, abnormal pupil size or response, irrational behaviour, sweating, or absence of sweating (overheating disorder), agitation, seizures, unsteady on feet or staggering walk, heavy smell of alcohol on a patient's breath, tremor, breathing difficulty, evidence of a suicide note, evidence of empty bottles or containers by the patient.

chapter fifteen: bites and stings

1. a) Preventing further envenomation.
   b) Pain management.
   c) Resuscitation, as necessary.
2. a) Snake bite: Pressure-immobilisation bandaging.
   b) Stingray barb: Heat treatment.
   c) Minor *Chironex* sting: Vinegar.
   d) Funnel-web spider: Pressure-immobilisation bandaging.
   e) Red-back spider: Cold treatment.
   f) Cone shells: Pressure-immobilisation bandaging.
3. Ice massage is appropriate if a sting covers a large area, particularly if the patient is cold or wet, and using cold therapy over a large area may cause hypothermia.
4. Vinegar used for a minimum of 30 seconds prevents further stinging from tentacles that may remain on the skin after a *Chironex* box jellyfish sting. Vinegar does not reduce pain and does not reverse the effects of venom already injected.
5. Pressure-immobilisation bandaging delays absorption of venom from the affected area, thereby delaying the onset of symptoms.
6. a) Breathing problems.
   b) Heart irregularity.
   c) Loss of consciousness.
   d) The sting covers more than half of one limb.
7. Any five of the following: severe backache, muscle cramps, anxiety, restlessness, sweating, nausea, headache, a 'feeling of impending doom', hypertension.

chapter sixteen: temperature-related illness and injury

1. b.
2. Mild forms of frostbite affect only the skin, and usually recover well, however, severe frostbite affects deeper tissues, including blood vessels, which deprives the area of oxygen, usually resulting in permanent damage, tissue death and gangrene.
3. d.
4. d.
5. Any five of the following: painful limb cramps, stomach cramps, excessive sweating, thirst, fatigue or dizziness, nausea, vomiting.
6. The skin feels hot and dry because the sweating mechanism is switched off as the body attempts to stop the loss of fluid. People become restless or aggressive, confused, disoriented and may experience seizures or lose consciousness.
7. a) Superficial burns.
   b) Partial-thickness burns.
   c) Full-thickness burns.
8. a) Unconsciousness.
   b) Confusion.
   c) Burns to skin, with (usually) an entry and an exit point.
   d) Irregular, weak or absent pulse.
9. Stop, drop and roll. Stop the patient from running, cover them in a (non-synthetic) blanket, or similar, to smother the flames, lay them on the ground and roll them until the flames have been extinguished.
10. b.

chapter seventeen: hard and soft tissue injuries

1. a) Fractures.
   b) Dislocations.
   c) Subluxations.
2. An open fracture may be caused by bone piercing the skin and soft tissue when it breaks, or from an object penetrating the skin and fracturing a bone. A closed fracture is more common and occurs when the skin remains intact (unbroken).
3. a) Loss of function.
   b) Swelling at the site.
   c) Deformity.
   d) Unnatural movement.
   e) Shock.
4. A dislocation is an injury in which a bone is moved out of its normal position in relation to another bone with which it forms a joint. Subluxations are incomplete dislocations. Treatment is the same.
5. A strain is a simple soft tissue injury affecting muscle, and is usually caused by overstretching. Strains will usually heal by themselves, though there may be complications if tendons are involved.
6. a) Swelling.
   b) Loss of power or ability to bear weight.
   c) Possible discolouration.
   d) Sudden-onset pain.
7. R: Rest. Have the injured person rest the injured part.
   I: Ice. Use ice or a cold pack (covered with a cloth) to reduce pain and swelling.
   C: Compression. Wrap a compression bandage around the injured area, preferably over the ice pack.
   E: Elevation. Raise the affected area above the level of the heart.
   R: Referral. Refer the casualty to an appropriate health care professional for definitive diagnosis and continuing management.
8. a) H: Heat. Avoid all sources of heat, which will increase blood supply and bruising.
   b) A: Alcohol. Consuming alcohol may increase swelling.
   c) R: Running. Exercising the area too soon may aggravate and worsen the injury. Only contusions should be stretched or gently exercised some hours after the injury.
   d) M: Massage. Any form of massage to the area will increase blood flow and bruising.

chapter eighteen: moving injured casualties

1. In the absence of medical help, moving a casualty should only be attempted when the patient is in immediate or imminent danger, as any movement may worsen their injury.
2. Any five of the following: danger, location, route of movement, equipment, personnel, urgency, safe methods of lifting and carrying.
3. a) Scoop.
   b) Spinal board.
   c) Blankets.
4. a) One-person human crutch.
   b) Two-person human crutch.
   c) Two-handed seat.
   d) Four-handed seat.
   e) Emergency drags.
5. 3 Ask the patient to place their arms around the first aiders' necks.
   5 First aiders should stand at the same time and start walking with the outside leg.
   1 Two first aiders stand facing each other behind the patient.
   2 Each first aider holds their own left wrist and grasps the other person's right wrist with their left hand creating the 'seat'.
   4 Squatting down, bring the four-handed seat under the patient.

chapter nineteen: drug and substance abuse

1. Drug and substance abuse includes the abuse and overdose of illicit, prescription and non-prescription medication and other substances in a manner not intended by the manufacturer or in doses above those directed.
2. Any five of the following: increase alertness and mask the signs of fatigue, produce feelings of euphoria and increased well-being, cause anxiety and bizarre behaviour, increase heart rate, increase blood pressure, increase respiratory rate, dilation of pupils, suppress appetite, insomnia.
3. a) Caffeine.
   b) Nicotine.
   c) Amphetamines.
   d) Cocaine.
   e) Crack.
4. Any five of the following: analgesia, anaesthesia, decrease heart rate, decrease respiratory rate, relief from anxiety, sedation, produce feelings of euphoria and increased well-being.
5. a) Alcohol.
   b) Narcotic analgesics.
   c) General anaesthetics.
   d) Sedative hypnotics.
   e) Cannabis.
6. Any five of the following: marijuana/hashish (a depressant at low doses), LSD (lysergic acid diethylamide), mescaline, psylocybin, PCP (phenylcyclidine), ecstasy.

chapter twenty: emergency childbirth

1. a) Calling for an ambulance.
   b) Protecting the mother and child from infection.
   c) Assisting with the birth of the baby.
   d) Caring for the newborn infant.
   e) Delivery of the placenta.
2. a) Early phase.
   b) Active phase.
   c) Transition.
3. During stage 1 labour, the cervix effaces, or thins out and dilates to 10 cm to allow the baby's head to descend into the vagina for delivery. Full dilation and effacement of the cervix marks the end of stage 1 labour and the beginning of stage 2.
4. b.
5. A breech birth occurs when a body part other than the head appears first — feet or buttocks are the most common.

chapter twenty-one: spinal injuries and management

1. With proper management, if the spinal cord has not been severed or damaged on the initial impact, it can be protected against further trauma. Unless an accident has been witnessed or if a spinal injury is highly improbable, always treat motionless and unconscious patients for a spinal injury.
2. a) Vertical compression.
   b) Flexion with rotation.
3. a) Back or neck pain.
   b) Tingling or lack of feeling in lower or upper limbs.
   c) Increased muscle tone.
   d) Dizziness.
   e) Headache.
4. Casualties found lying in awkward or unusual positions should not be moved unless under the supervision of an experienced rescue and/or pre-hospital worker with specific equipment, unless they are at risk of danger.
5. a) Managing airway and circulation.
   b) Minimising movement of the head and cervical spine.
   c) Minimising movement of the thoracic and lumbar spine, sacrum and coccyx.

chapter twenty-two: triage

1. Triage is the initial assessment and sorting of patients based on medical need and likely response to treatment.
2. a) To prioritise treatment to use available resources as efficiently as possible.
   b) To ensure care is focused on those patients most likely to benefit from the limited resources available.
   c) To provide a framework for difficult and stressful life-and-death decisions.
   d) To create order in a chaotic environment.
3. a) Ensure the airway is open.
   b) Control major bleeds.
   c) Elevate the legs.
4. Patients with life-threatening but treatable injuries, requiring immediate medical attention. These patients are the first to be transported to hospital when medical help arrives, without delaying transportation for stabilisation.
5. Patients with serious injuries, but able to wait a short time for treatment.
6. Patients who can wait hours to days for treatment. These patients can be separated from the more seriously injured by asking for patients able to walk (i.e. 'minor' patients) to congregate in a specified area.
7. The START triage system classifies a patient's treatment category from an assessment of their respiratory, circulatory and neurological function. Patients are then attributed to one of the following four categories: 'immediate', 'urgent', 'delayed' or 'dead'.

chapter twenty-three: advanced resuscitation and oxygen administration

1. Any five of the following: unconsciousness, shock, blood loss, chest pain, shortness of breath, circulatory distress, severe pain, injuries, after resuscitation.
2. c.
3. A full 'C' cylinder (440–490 L) will have the following approximate operational times:
   - 50 minutes, with continuous use of oxygen therapy at ~8 L per minute
   - 30 minutes, with continuous use of airbag (and oxygen) at ~14–15 L per minute.
4. OP airways are curved plastic devices that help keep the airway clear in the unconscious patient by depressing the tongue and keeping the teeth and lips apart.
5. The distance between the lips and the angle of the jaw.
6. d.

chapter twenty-four: defibrillation

1. Defibrillation is the delivery of an electric shock to revert the heart to its normal (sinus) rhythm in the event of specific cardiac arrhythmias.
2. The heart's pacemaker cells, or sinoatrial node, are located in the wall of the right atrium. After spreading through the atria, electrical impulses continue down to the atrioventricular node in the ventricles, causing them to contract.

3. N   Asystole.
   Y   Ventricular fibrillation.
   Y   Pulseless ventricular tachycardia.
   N   Sinus rhythm.
4. a) The patient is unresponsive.
   b) The patient is not breathing.
   c) The patient has no pulse.
   d) The first aider has access to an SAED.
   e) The first aider is trained/certified in the use of the SAED.
5. a) Place the sternum electrode pad to the right of the sternum (breastbone) below the collarbone and above the right nipple.
   b) Place the apex electrode pad to the left of the sternum, with the upper edge of the pad below and to the left of the nipple.
6. d.

chapter twenty-five: pain management and administration of analgesic gases

1. Whether applying simple methods such as ice, or formal pain management techniques, the principles are the same — relieve the patient's suffering, as you are unlikely to be able to stop the pain.
2. a) Reassurance.
   b) Cold packs for local skin pain.
   c) Heat for penetrating marine injuries.
   d) Administration of nitrous oxide or methoxyflurane for severe pain.
3. Entonox is a mixture of 50% nitrous oxide and 50% oxygen.
4. Any five of the following: the casualty cannot understand or comply with instructions for use, suspected air embolus, suspected decompression sickness, suspected pneumothorax, suspected bowel obstruction, decreased level of consciousness, impaired gas exchange.
5. a) Nausea and vomiting.
   b) Dizziness.
   c) Drowsiness.
   d) Temporary loss of consciousness.
6. a) History of kidney disease (renal impairment or renal failure).
   b) Head injury or an altered state of consciousness from any cause (including alcohol).
   c) Respiratory depression.
   d) Cardiovascular instability.
7. a) Nausea.
   b) Vomiting.
   c) Headache.
   d) Skin irritation.
8. a) Profound respiratory and circulatory depression.
   b) Loss of consciousness.
   c) Severe kidney disease.

glossary

Acidity The quality or extent of being acid, as of gastric juices, which neutralise alkalis

Adrenal glands Situated on the superior surface of the kidneys, involved in the control of main body systems

Adrenaline An important hormone secreted by the adrenal gland, which has the function of preparing the body for fight or flight and has widespread effects throughout the autonomic nervous system

Aerobic (exercise) Relating to physical exercise which stimulates the respiratory and circulatory systems to improve and maintain physical fitness, intending to increase oxygen consumption and to benefit the lungs and cardiovascular system

Alkalinity The quality or extent of being alkaline, which neutralises acids

Ambient Completely surrounding or circulating around, as in atmosphere or fluid

Amniotic fluid The fluid contained within the amniotic cavity surrounding the growing foetus (baby)

Anaesthesia Loss of feeling in all or part of a body. The term is usually applied to the technique of reducing or abolishing pain to enable surgery to be performed. May be 'local' — limited to an area — or 'general' — involving the whole body

Analgesia Reduced sensibility to pain, without loss of consciousness and without the sense of touch necessarily being affected. It may occur accidentally or be induced deliberately by the use of pain-killing drugs

Anaphylaxis An abnormal (sometimes allergic) reaction of the body to an antigen whereby histamine is produced and released, which may cause an extreme and generalised allergic reaction resulting in swelling, constriction of bronchioles, heart failure, circulatory collapse and, sometimes, death

Angina The pain associated with restricted blood supply to the heart muscle. It is often felt as a suffocating pain in the centre of the chest, often induced by exercise and relieved by rest, which may spread to the jaw or radiate down the arms

Anxiety Generalised pervasive fear, where a patient's life and thoughts are dominated by fear

Antigens Foreign substance the body sees as potentially dangerous

Arrhythmia Any deviation from the normal (sinus) rhythm of the heart

Asystole Condition in which the heart no longer beats, accompanied by the absence of electrical activity in the heart, as shown on an electrocardiogram, showing cardiac arrest

Atherosclerosis The build-up of fatty plaques in arterial walls restricting blood flow to distal tissues. Unstable plaques may rupture, causing a blood clot (thrombus), which may dislodge and block an artery at another site (thromboembolism)

Atrioventricular node A mass of specialised heart muscle situated in the lower middle part of the right atrium, which receives the impulse to contract from the sinoatrial node and transmits it through to the ventricles to cause them to contract as part of a heartbeat

Avulsion The tearing or forcible separation of part of a structure (e.g. tooth avulsion). Severe avulsions are equivalent to amputations (e.g. finger avulsion, limb avulsion)

Barbituate A class of sedative/hypnotic drugs that depress the activity of the central nervous system

Basal metabolism The minimum amount of energy expended by the body to maintain vital processes, e.g. respiration, circulation and digestion

Benzodiazepines A class of sedative/hypnotic drugs that depress the activity of the central nervous system (tranquillisers)

Braxton-Hicks (contractions) Painless contractions of the uterus more common towards the end of pregnancy preparing the uterus for delivery

Bronchospasm Narrowing of bronchi (in the lungs) by muscular contraction in response to some stimulus as in asthma and bronchitis. The patient can usually inhale air into the lungs, but exhalation may require visible muscular effort and may be accompanied by wheezing

Cerebral Relating to the cerebrum, or right and left cerebral hemispheres, which are connected by fibre pathways (commissures), e.g. cerebral haemorrhage — bleeding from a cerebral artery into the brain

Cerebrovascular disease The build-up of fatty plaques (atherosclerosis) restricting blood flow to the brain resulting in stroke or haemorrhage

Cervix The neck-like part of the uterus that opens into the vagina

Clonic Term used to describe the jerking limb movements in convulsive epilepsy, as in tonic clonic seizures

Concussion A limited period of unconsciousness or reduced consciousness caused by injury to the head. There may be no recognisable structural damage to the brain

Contusion Also called a bruise. An area of skin discolouration caused by the escape of blood from ruptured underlying vessels following injury. A contusion may also affect the brain after a head injury

Cornea The transparent dome-shaped tissue covering the iris, pupil and lens. The cornea contains no blood vessels and it is extremely sensitive to pain

Crowning The stage of labour when the infant's head is visible at the vaginal opening

Cyanosed When a person has a bluish discolouration of the skin and mucous membranes resulting from an inadequate amount of oxygen in the blood. It may also be seen in babies (so called blue babies) because of heart defects

Dander Scales from animal skins, hair or feathers that can be potent allergens

Delusional Someone who has irrationally-held beliefs that cannot be altered by rational argument

Dentures Removable replacement for one or more teeth carried on some type of plate or frame

Dermis The thick layer of living tissue that lies beneath the epidermis (outer layer of skin)

Dilate (childbirth) The enlargement of the cervix to 10 cm during the first stage of labour, which in conjunction with effacement, allows the baby to descend into the vagina during delivery

Dislocation Displacement of bones from their normal position in a joint

Dousing To drench or plunge into water or like

Duodenum The first of the three parts of the small intestine, which receives bile from the gall bladder and pancreatic juices from the pancreas

Efface (childbirth) The term used to describe the thinning out of the cervix during the first stage of labour, which in conjunction with dilation, allows the baby to descend into the vagina during delivery

Electrolytes A solution containing salts/ions, which can be easily administered by mouth or intravenous drip to correct seriously diminished electrolyte levels and dehydration in a patient

Embolus Material, such as a blood clot, fat, air or a foreign body, that is carried by the blood from one point in the circulation to lodge at another point

Envenomation To be impregnated with venom, made poisonous

Epidermis The outer layer of the skin

Erythroxylon (coca bush) Bush from which cocaine is derived

Euphoria A state of optimism, cheerfulness and well-being

Exacerbate To aggravate, irritate or make worse

Flexion The bending of a joint so that the angle between the bones of a joint is decreased

Ganglia Bundles of nerve cells outside the brain and spine

Haemorrhage A discharge of blood, as from a ruptured blood vessel, to bleed severely or violently

Hallucinogen A drug that produces hallucinations, e.g. cannabis and LSD

Hemisphere (cerebral) One of the two halves of the cerebrum — the largest part of the brain

Homeopathy A system of medicine based on the theory that 'like cures like'. The patient is treated with extremely small quantities of drugs that are themselves capable of producing symptoms of the particular disease

Hypercholesterolaemia An elevation of cholesterol in the blood. Cholesterol is a fat-like material synthesised in the liver and consumed in the diet. Cholesterol is present in the blood and most tissue, especially nervous tissues, and is an important constituent of hormones

Hyperglycaemia An excess of sugar in the bloodstream

Hypertension High blood pressure, an elevation of the arterial blood pressure above the normal range expected in a particular age group

Hyperventilation Breathing at an abnormally rapid rate at rest causing a reduction in carbon dioxide concentration in the blood

Hypoglycaemia A deficiency of sugar in the bloodstream

Hypotension A condition where the blood pressure is abnormally low

Hypoventilation Breathing at an abnormally shallow and slow rate causing an increase in carbon dioxide concentration in the blood

Hypoxia Deficiency of oxygen in the tissues

Immunoglobulin One of a group of structurally related proteins that act as antibodies

Impact To firmly wedge, e.g. an impacted fracture is one in which the bone ends are driven into each other

Implicit Virtually contained

Inco-ordination An impairment in the performance of precise movement

Intercostal (muscles) Muscles that occupy the spaces between the ribs, which are responsible for movement of the ribs

Iris The coloured musculature in the front of the eye that regulates the amount of light entering the eye by changing the diameter of the pupil

Irrigate Washing out a wound or hollow organ with a continuous flow of water or saline solution

Labour The sequence of actions by which a baby and placenta are expelled from the uterus at childbirth

Lumen The space within a tubular or sac-like part, such as a blood vessel, the intestine or the stomach

Lymph A fluid present within the vessels of the lymphatic system, consisting of the fluid that bathes the tissues, which is derived from the blood and is drained by the lymphatic vessels

Mescaline An alkaloid present in the dried tops of Mexican cactus that causes inebriation and vivid colourful hallucinations when ingested

Metabolism The sum of the processes or chemical changes in an organism or a single cell by which nutrients from the blood are broken down with the exchange of energy

Myocardial infarction Death of a segment of heart muscle, which follows interruption of its blood supply

Neurological Relating to the structure, functioning and diseases of the nervous system

Nociceptors Nerve fibres, endings or pathways that are concerned with the perception of pain

Occlusion The closing or obstruction of a hollow organ or part

Optimum The best or most favourable point, degree or amount

Orifice A mouth-like opening or hole

Otitis media An infection of the middle ear

Pallor Abnormal paleness of the skin due to reduced blood flow or lack of normal pigments

Palpable Readily or plainly felt, that can be touched, e.g. to palpate a pulse, is to feel for it over a major artery

Paradoxical respirations Breathing movement in which the chest wall moves in on inspiration and out on expiration, in reverse of the normal movements

Paranoid Describing a mental state characterised by fixed and logically elaborate delusions of persecution or grandeur

Percussion (obstruction) The technique of tapping (with adequate pressure) on a patient's back between their shoulder blades with the intention of dislodging an obstruction in the airway

Perfused The passage of fluid through a vessel. Usually refers to blood and oxygen supply to tissues

Perineum The region of the body between the anus and the urethral/vaginal opening, including the skin and underlying muscle

Peripheral Outside of ..., external to ...

Perpendicular Meeting a given line or surface at right angles (i.e. at 90 degrees)

Pituitary gland The master endocrine gland in the brain, which secretes hormones that regulate many bodily functions

Placenta A vascular structure, which develops during pregnancy to provide the embryo with nourishment, eliminate its wastes and exchange respiratory gases

Pneumothorax Any breach of the lung surface or chest wall that allows air to enter the pleural cavity (gap between the two layers of covering of the lungs) causing the lungs to collapse

Prone Lying with the face downwards with the forearms in a position in which the palms are face downwards

Psychosis One of a group of mental disorders that feature loss of contact with reality

Saline A salt solution containing sodium chloride

Sinoatrial node The pacemaker of the heart, a microscopic area of specialised cardiac muscle located in the upper wall of the right atrium

Sinus rhythm A normal heart rhythm

Stridor The noise heard on breathing when the trachea or larynx is obstructed, it tends to be louder and harsher than a wheeze

Subluxation Partial dislocation of a joint so that the bone ends are misaligned, but still in contact

Swab A pad of absorbent material

Syncope Fainting, loss of consciousness induced by a temporarily insufficient flow of blood to the brain

Thyroid gland A large endocrine gland situated in the base of the neck

Tonic Term used to describe the muscle stiffening in convulsive epilepsy, as in tonic clonic seizures

Toxicity The degree to which a substance is poisonous

Umbilical cord The tissue connecting the foetus to the placenta containing two arteries and one vein

Vascular Relating to, or supplied with blood vessels

Ventricles Either of the two lower chambers of the heart

Ventricular fibrillation (VF) Rapid and chaotic beating of the heart rendering it unable to effectively pump blood throughout the body, which may result in cardiac arrest

Ventricular tachycardia (VT) An abnormally rapid heart rate, such that normal distribution of blood throughout the body is severely compromised. Typically causes breathlessness and possibly heart failure

Visceral Referring to the organs within the body cavities, especially the organs of the abdominal cavity

index

permissions

p 60   Identification bracelet/necklace © MedicAlert Australia
p 63   Hyperbaric chamber © Wesley Centre for Hyperbaric Medicine
p 107 Red-back spider © Lochman Transparencies
p 108 Sydney funnel web spider © DW Stock Picture Library
p 108 Tiger snake © Lochman Transparencies
p 109 Paralysis tick © DW Stock Picture Library, Holt Studios
p 159 Waterfall train disaster © Newspix